Why Me? Why Anyone?

Why Me? Why Anyone?

Hirshel Jaffe,
James Rudin, and Marcia Rudin

St. Martin's Press
New York

WHY ME? WHY ANYONE?
Copyright © 1986 by Hirshel Jaffe, James Rudin, and Marcia Rudin. All rights reserved. Printed in the United States of America. No part of this book may be used or reproduced in any manner whatsoever without written permission except in the case of brief quotations embodied in critical articles or reviews. For information, address St. Martin's Press, 175 Fifth Avenue, New York, N.Y. 10010.

Library of Congress Cataloging in Publication Data
Jaffe, Hirshel.
    Why me? Why anyone?
      1. Jaffe, Hirshel—Health.   2. Rabbis—New York
(State)—Newburgh—Biography.   3. Leukemia—Patients—
Biography.   I. Rudin, A. James (Arnold James),
1934– .   II. Rudin, Marcia R., 1940– .
III. Title.
BM755.J25A38 1986   296.7'4   85-26060
ISBN 0-312-87803-6

First Edition

10 9 8 7 6 5 4 3 2 1

For Judith Anne Jaffe

Acknowledgments

We owe so much to the physicians and nurses and other members of the hospital staffs for their healing and compassion. Thanks also to the Jaffes' friends in Dallas, and the congregants of Temple Beth Jacob in Newburgh, New York, for their warm support.

A thank-you to the staffs of the libraries of the American Jewish Committee and the Hebrew Union College–Jewish Institute of Religion in New York City for their assistance in locating materials. Our appreciation to Rabbi Maurice Lamm, who helped clarify some points concerning Judaism's position on bio-ethical issues, and to Florence Mordhorst and Elaine Gerstein for their technical assistance.

Our agent, Berenice Hoffman, strongly believed in this project from the very beginning, and without her guidance and support we could not have written this book. For her patience and wisdom we thank her.

Very special praise for Joyce Engelson, our amazingly perceptive, wonderful editor, whose constant insistence on excellence spurred us on to do our very best.

And, finally, we thank our combined total of four daughters, Rachel and Nina Jaffe and Eve and Jennifer Rudin, for their always-honest and refreshing criticisms.

Why Me?
Why Anyone?

1

My best friend, Hirshel Jaffe, has leukemia.
I found out a few days ago, and I still can't believe it.

We have been rabbis and friends for more than twenty years, and in all that time I've never seen Hirshel sick or even tired. He had boundless energy, always in perpetual motion, never still. He could play three sets of tennis on the hottest day and later go out and run six miles to channel his enormous natural enthusiasm and nervous energy. Running was his real passion. Even Hirshel's Hebrew name, Zvi, means "deer" or "swift runner."

I'll never forget the day he ran in the New York City Marathon.

It was a beautiful late October afternoon in 1978, so warm that the marathon participants were complaining. I was in Central Park with my wife, Marcia, and our two daughters, watching thousands of long-distance runners cross the finish line after their grueling twenty-six-mile course had touched each of New York City's five boroughs. But we were really there to cheer on our good friend Hirshel. He had been training for ten years. How many miles he must have run to prepare for this day!

Although jammed in a huge crowd, by some miracle we saw Hirshel bounding toward the finish line. He was sporting a T-shirt with bold blue-and-white letters proclaiming him "The Running Rabbi." Amazingly, it seemed as if he had energy to spare even after running twenty-six miles. Hirshel was smiling triumphantly, and as he ran across the finish line we could hear him shout, "I did it! I did it!"

Hirshel paced back and forth to cool his body down gradually. One of the marathon officials threw a silver foil insulating cape around him to prevent his body heat from escaping too quickly. Hirshel's wife, Judi, and their children, Nina and Rachel, ran over to him and threw their arms around their personal champion.

We all walked together and sat down under a large tree. I urged Hirshel to lie down in the shade and rest, but he said, "No, I'm fine. I'm hardly tired, Jim. I feel so great I think I could run the whole thing all over again."

We laughed as Hirshel started to nibble on the snack food provided to all who finished the grueling race. Little groups of exhausted but happy runners and their admiring families and friends were scattered, some standing, some sitting, all over the Sheep Meadow in Central Park. The rays of the bright autumn sun reflected off the hundreds of silver capes. The runners reminded me of medieval knights in their shining armor, resting after a long and strenuous battle. "I did it, I did it! I made it!" Hirshel repeated over and over again, as if he couldn't believe it. He was beaming.

Now, less than three years later, that same tall, trim, highly conditioned body is out of control, wracked by insidious killer cancer cells Hirshel Jaffe didn't even know about until it was almost too late. My active, aggressive, energetic friend—only forty-six years old—always so forceful and in such control of his own life, is now waiting in a hospital, at the mercy of physicians and a medical technology that may not be able to help him.

The first hint Marcia and I received that something was wrong with Hirshel came only a few weeks ago. The Jaffe family was spending the day with us at our vacation home in the Poconos. Our favorite pizza place was closed, so we all had dinner that night at a family restaurant we had never eaten in before. Our mistake. The food was terrible, but we were managing to gag it down until Judi found a dead fly in her baked potato. After we got over the shock and stopped laughing we called the waitress over to show her the fly. She went to get the manager. When we complained to the manager, he said he wasn't responsible for the dead fly in the potato. "God must have put it there," he conjectured. However, he did subtract fifty-nine cents, the estimated cost of the potato, from our total bill.

We were still talking about the incident as we walked out to our cars, but when I casually asked Hirshel if he'd been playing any good tennis lately, he said, "No, I don't have enough energy for both tennis and running." His answer caught Marcia and me by surprise. It was so unlike Hirshel to have to ration his energy. He has always been so healthy and vigorous. And we noticed a slight edge in his voice. Little did we know that that very morning, when he and Judi picked up their girls from camp, he could hardly walk in the heat and couldn't carry the children's trunks.

Tomorrow the doctors are going to take out Hirshel's spleen. Marcia and I and our daughters, Eve and Jennifer, have traveled to the hospital to visit him and to cheer him on, just as we cheered him over the marathon finish line that sunny day that now seems so long ago. But, I ask myself, what can I say to Hirshel today that will cheer him? Will I be able to give him the emotional support he's going to need? I'm one of his best friends, so if I can't help him, who can?

3

As a rabbi, Hirshel Jaffe has always been there to comfort others when they need it. But who will comfort Hirshel? Who will be his rabbi? Hirshel has always been like a shepherd to his flock of congregants. Who will be Hirshel's shepherd now?

Most of us turn to our religion in times of emotional crisis because it provides meaning to our lives and helps us. Will our Jewish tradition bring solace to my friend? I wonder. Will all the things he has been telling his congregants, when they come to him with their agonizing pain, comfort Hirshel now that *he* is the one that needs it? Or will he find the words we rabbis have learned to say over the years just glib, empty clichés?

I spot Hirshel at the end of the hospital corridor. He is wearing cutoff pajamas, a short bathrobe, bright sweat socks, and his well-worn Nike running shoes. His incongruous outfit makes me laugh. But as he walks toward me, my amusement fades when I see how pale he is. He's lost a lot of weight, which makes him look even taller and more gaunt than usual, and makes his dark-brown mustache seem too large for his face.

Hirshel grasps my hand and steers me toward his hospital room. "Jim, so good to see you!" He is smiling, obviously trying to be cheerful. But behind his heavy tortoiseshell glasses his eyes have a haunted look, a look of desperation. Like the look in the eyes of my brother, Bert, when he realized he was going to die of his Hodgkin's disease. I'll never forget those eyes. Hirshel has them now. My brother had his spleen removed also in a vain attempt to stop his cancer. This whole scenario is agonizingly familiar to me.

Hirshel has tried to make the room cheerful. There are dozens of cards and bouquets of flowers from his congregants at Temple Beth Jacob in Newburgh, New York. He's very well-known and liked, and the news of his illness has shaken the synagogue and the community. Above his bed he's taped a photo of himself finishing the 1978 New York Marathon in his "Running Rabbi" T-shirt. Nearby is a giant funny card some congregants made to cheer him up. On the other wall are pictures of Judi and the children. Judi has put up a *Playboy* pinup, X-rated cartoons, and Murphy's famous law that proclaims, "When one things starts to go wrong, everything will go wrong." Judi, a nurse, knows about mix-ups in hospitals.

But no matter how many cards and flowers fill a patient's little space, no matter how humorous the pinups and comforting the mementos from home, hospital rooms are always grim. As a rabbi I have been visiting patients for twenty-five years, and I know the rooms are always somehow the same. They're hot and stuffy, and stale odors left over from a thousand unappetizing and often uneaten meals hang in the air.

Trying to hide my discomfort, I smile as I sit down on the hard chair next to his bed.

"You look good, Hirshel," I begin, lying a little.

"I'm very up, Jim. A little nervous, of course. I've never had surgery before. Now I just want to get it over with. The doctors said it's a routine operation. 'A piece of cake,' they told me. My blood count is dangerously low now, but it should bounce back right after the spleen comes out. So you know me, Jim, I'm an up person, and I feel hopeful."

"Tell me what happened, Hirshel. We're still so confused. When did you find out . . . ?"

"It all happened so fast, Jim, that's what's so unbelievable. Suddenly I started to feel really fatigued and listless. That was the beginning of July—about a month ago. Weary, hardly any energy. I felt sleepy in the middle of the day, and sometimes I had to leave the temple and go home to lie down. And I couldn't run as far or as fast as usual. My running buddies started to notice. I tried to keep running, but the hills felt like mountains to me. I was fighting sleep at the wheel of my jeep, and I was afraid I'd have an accident. I just felt so drained.

"I complained to Judi about how bad I felt. And finally in her blunt, direct way she said, 'You better go to the doctor, Hirshel, it could be something very serious.' But I still didn't make an appointment.

"One day a friend flew me in his plane up to Martha's Vineyard for the day so I could check on our summer house. We went running on the beach, and when we were finished I noticed a bruise on my ankle. I knew I hadn't fallen down or hurt it—I had just been running as usual. I was really scared because the bruise was such a visible sign. Like a stigma. And I couldn't shake the fatigue. Finally I asked a friend to recommend an internist. You know, Jim, I didn't even have a doctor. I hadn't been to one in years.

"Well, the internist wasn't too concerned at first about my fatigue, but I pushed him to give me a blood test. The counts came out really low. He must have been hoping for a simple explanation like mononucleosis or a virus, but I knew my body well enough to sense something was very wrong. My blood counts kept dropping, and they kept redoing the tests. Meanwhile I started nervously scanning Judi's medical textbooks to see if I could find out what was wrong.

"The internist knew we were leaving soon for our month on Martha's Vineyard, and he said, 'Rabbi, why don't you go on your vacation? I'll see you in a month. You should bounce back.' But I said, 'No, I don't want to go away not knowing what's the matter.' Then he said very quietly and seriously, as if he knew I thought I had cancer, 'All right, we'll look further. Let's examine your bone marrow.'

"They didn't see anything abnormal in the bone marrow biopsy, but by now my blood count was alarmingly low. My fears grew when the internist called and said, 'Rabbi, we want you nearby where we can watch you. Maybe it would be better to postpone your trip.'

"But they still weren't coming up with a diagnosis. Luckily I have a friend who's a pathologist, and he said, 'Why don't you come up to my lab and let me take a look at your blood?'

"There was my friend peering through his electron microscope. He told me later he saw the weird-looking cancer cell growing in me from his very first look. His mind must have been racing, but he was trying to carry it off calmly. He asked me if anyone had examined my spleen. I didn't realize the significance of his question at the time. He called a hematologist friend. Judi and I sat in the hematologist's office a few days ago and heard everything confirmed. I have hairy-cell leukemia."

"Harry?"

"H-a-i-r-y. Like on your head. The cells looks like a hair under a microscope. That's how the disease got its name. They don't know much about it. It's very rare. There are only about two hundred cases a year in the United States, less than two percent of all leukemias, the physicians told me. So here I am, Jim, the indestructible Hirshel Jaffe, never sick a day in my life. My spleen is very enlarged, and that's dangerous so they have to get it out. A spleenectomy is the first step in battling this strange leukemia. I dread surgery, but I have to have it. We'll lick this! We'll use every medical technique we have. Do I have any choice?"

"Will they give you chemotherapy after the surgery?"

"No. Aggressive chemotherapy doesn't seem to help hairy-cell leukemia. The doctors explained that they don't like to do anything except take out the spleen until absolutely necessary because sometimes the disease can be chronic and progress very slowly."

"Are your parents here, Hirshel?"

"No, they're still up in our house on the Vineyard. Why should they break up their vacation? It's a long trip. And my doctor said I'll be up there in a week and they can see me there. I can recuperate lying on our deck watching the surf. . . . By the way, we really appreciate you and Marcia taking our girls this week. It gives Judi a chance to breathe and visit me. I can't thank you enough. I realize now how much it means to have friends who care about you."

"Didn't you already know that?"

"I guess it never came home to me before that I needed anybody that much. I was always worrying about everyone else's problems. Now for a change I have to worry about myself. I still haven't gotten over the shock of the diagnosis yet. A lot of things are racing through my mind. I am thinking, 'My God, you're vulnerable, Hirshel, you've really got something wrong with you.'

"I thought I'd always have my perfect health. You know me, Jim, I've always had so much energy. I was running six or seven miles a day. It became my second religion. My body was conditioned so well it responded to all my demands. I always ate the right food, never smoked or drank except for wine on Shabbas. Judi used to tease me about my health fetishes.

"I guess I thought if I jogged I'd live forever. I remember once, about two years ago, I made a kind of bargain with God. I was feeling great, running alone on South Beach in front of our house on Martha's Vineyard. The surf was awesome. It was a gorgeous day. I could run six or eight miles in the wet sand right on the edge of the water and keep up with those high school track athletes training there. I was feeling indestructible, and I looked up to the heavens and said, 'Hey, I'm going to live to be one hundred and twenty, maybe more.' I was saying, 'Well, God, I'll just take care of my body. You want human beings to be healthy, don't you?' "

"Pacts with God can be dangerous, Hirshel."

"It wasn't really a Faustian bargain because I didn't agree to give very much back to God. I was just being selfish. I felt so triumphant. You know, the *Rocky* image. The waves were coming in, and there were lovers on the beach, and I'm thinking I'll push death away.

"For years Judi's been trying to warn me. She said, 'Hirshel, with all your running, you think you're going to live forever? You could get a stroke or cancer, anything can happen.' I used to get so angry at her I'd go out and run ten more miles. All the while she was saying to me, 'Hirshel, don't think you're indestructible.' Well, now I've discovered she was right. Judi is so right about nearly everything."

"I'd feel indestructible too, Hirshel, if I were in your shape. You're young, lots of life ahead of you. We never expect anything like this to happen to us. It always happens to somebody else. God, why does it have to be you? It's just not fair. I would be so angry!"

"I'm really not angry, Jim. Maybe being a rabbi makes me more accepting because I deal with illness all the time. That's part of my job. I know I can't will or wish away this disease. Besides, it won't do me any good to be angry."

"I don't know. Maybe it would make you feel better if you got angry. Do you feel guilty instead?" Am I being tactless in asking my friend this question? I wonder. But I push ahead anyway. "You know, Hirshel, some people

9

feel guilty when they find out they're sick. That's their first reaction, almost like a reflex. They think maybe God is punishing them for something they've done. One woman said to me years ago when her husband died, 'I guess I should have kept a kosher home.' I had another congregant who thought his daughter was killed because he had been cheating on his wife. He actually half-believed it. I told him I don't think God works like that. But do you think God is punishing *you*, Hirshel?" Is this the time or the place for questions like this? I wonder again. Probably I should stop asking these heavy questions, but I'm very curious about what Hirshel thinks now. We've struggled with these issues together for so long as rabbinical students and as rabbis.

"You mean do I think God has sent me this illness, like that restaurant manager's theory that He put the dead fly in Judi's baked potato? No, I don't think my illness is part of some divine plan. It can happen to anyone. Maybe it's just chance. I don't think I was fated to have leukemia. You know Jews don't believe in blind fate, Jim.

"My congregants have been asking me these questions for twenty years. I've always told them, 'God doesn't single out people because they've been good or bad. Illness is just part of human vulnerability.' Of course, I'm not all that calm about it. When I heard I had leukemia, half of me said, 'O.K., you've got it, who are you to complain?' Maybe that was the rabbi half of me who has seen so much illness and buried so many people and who knows this can happen to anyone. But the other half of me, the human side, was already screaming out to someone, something, maybe to God, to save me."

"But didn't you scream out, 'God damn it for bringing this on me,' or 'Damn God for letting this happen to me'?" I press. "Jim," I tell myself, "stop grilling Hirshel.

He probably hasn't even had time to think about these things yet. Don't sound so harsh. I should be more sensitive to his feelings. But maybe if I force him to confront these questions, he'll be able to express his anger, and that will help him. I am here to offer my support to Hirshel, and I don't want to fail him. I hope I'll know the right thing to do."

"No, I don't curse God, Jim. And I want to tell people that. I want to say to my congregants, 'All the things I've been telling you all these years are true. We don't curse God.'"

I think, "Well, Jim, I hope you're proud of yourself. You've managed to thoroughly depress your friend instead of cheering him up. Let's change the subject." I point down to his Nike running shoes. "You know, Hirshel, you look like an imprisoned jogger."

Hirshel laughs. "Yeah, these sneakers do look a little funny with my pajamas, don't they? I guess I'm just trying to cling to my 'Running Rabbi' image. I threw that picture into my suitcase to remind me of my better days. I've been out in the halls just pacing around. I can't stand being cooped up in this room. . . ."

My wife walks into the room. Marcia immediately sees how pale and thin Hirshel is, and our eyes meet. I know she's thinking of my brother too, remembering the doom in Bert's eyes the last time she saw him in his hospital room.

"I'd better leave now, Hirshel," I tell my friend. "They only allow one visitor at a time up here. We'll be thinking of you tomorrow. Everything will be fine. We'll call you a day or so after your operation when you'll feel like talking."

As I am leaving the room, Hirshel gets out of bed and hugs Marcia. They just stand there with their arms around each other, not saying a word for a very long time. Two human beings reaching out to each other for warmth, the desire of an ill and anxious person to touch someone to ease his fears.

Hirshel and Marcia are still embracing as I leave the stuffy room and walk down the hall toward the elevator.

~~~~~

August 3, 1982

The hospital food is lousy, but I ate dinner anyway. I won't be able to snack after midnight like I do at home because of the early-morning surgery.

Judi and Rachel and Nina went out to eat with Jim and Marcia and their girls. All my visitors have left. For the first time I am all alone in here.

Everything has happened so fast, I haven't had time to sort out my thoughts and feelings. So I have decided to get my experiences and thoughts down on tape. Like a diary. I've never done anything like this before—never had the time or patience to be very introspective. But now I want to record what's happening to me because I think that will help me deal with it.

This is such a totally strange experience for me. There are moments when I can't believe I am really seriously ill. I've never even had the flu. For twenty years I've been the rabbi calling on hospital patients. I've witnessed everybody else's illnesses. Over the years I've learned just what to say to patients and how long to stay with them. I knew when to listen and when to recite the appropriate psalm. But not for a single day in my entire life have I ever been hospitalized. I could always leave the hospital room, walk to an elevator, and go out and jog.

But now it's a whole new ball game. I'm on the other side of the bed. Even if I never have to worry about my illness again, I sense this is going to change me, because now I'll know what it is to be sick in a hospital. I know from now on I won't be so rushed when I visit people, like I'm checking them off a list. And I won't wait so long to get there.

I can already see this experience will make a big difference in my work. Last week after I knew my diagnosis, I had to conduct a funeral for a lovely woman in my congregation, a Holocaust survivor. I got through the ceremony, but I was dwelling on my own mortality. At the cemetery when her daughter threw dirt onto her grave I thought, "That could be Rachel or Nina doing that for me."

And I wonder how my congregants will react. What happens to a congregation when its rabbi is afflicted with a dread disease? They think a rabbi is like a representative of God; they might have trouble seeing me as less than perfect. I hope they will realize I'm not perfect and they'll accept me now as just another human being like themselves with troubles of his own.

When Talmudic scholars asked, "Who is eligible to lead the Jewish people?" they answered it must be someone who is like everyone else—fully involved in life, married, raising children, struggling, and suffering. A rabbi is not priestly or above it all. Our Jewish spiritual leaders have always lived and worked like other people, never isolating themselves from the routine, everyday aspects—both good and bad—of life. Rabbi Hillel said, "Do not separate yourself from the community."

My illness is certainly affecting my daughters' lives. I could see that Rachel and Nina were anxious to leave my room today when they were visiting me. They've never seen their daddy sick before. They were trying to act nonchalant and cheer me up, but this must be so frightening to them. They looked so beautiful in their summer dresses. Nina has an absolutely radiant face when she smiles, and Rachel is going to be a very pretty teenager.

They know something is wrong with Daddy's blood and that it's serious. Nina empathizes so much and lets you know how *she feels. She was with Judi and me in the hospital when they put my blood through the Coulter Counter. She saw the surprised look on the technicians' faces when my blood count registered so low, and she blurted out, "Is my daddy going to die?" We all just looked at each other. It was heartbreaking.*

Rachel is more laid-back, but I'm sure she is just as anxious as Nina is. She just doesn't express it. It will be good for them to stay at the Rudins' in the Poconos while I have the surgery. They'll be distracted there and have a good time, and they won't have to see me right away after the operation. That might be pretty scary for them.

Judi is so cool in tough situations. That's why she was such a good nurse in the trauma unit when we lived in Dallas. She's joking now as always. I know she's trying to keep my spirits up. But I can read the expression in her big dark eyes, and I can tell she's shaken. She can't hide it from me.

She's so unaffected and refreshing. Everything is either black or white with Judi. There are very few grays. She keeps me thinking straight. I've always known I could never bullshit Judi, even when we were dating. That's why I was drawn to her—she doesn't give in to others, she has her own strong values, she's her own person. I knew if things ever got rough I could depend on her because she's so strong. I hope I can draw on some of her strength now.

I'll need it.

2

~~~~~

We find a German restaurant near Hirshel's hospital. The food is too heavy for a hot summer day, and we aren't really hungry yet. But we want to eat early because Judi has an hour's drive to Newburgh and we have a long way back to the Poconos.

Judi is anxious to get the surgery out of the way. She's looking forward to taking Hirshel to Martha's Vineyard in a few days so she can have some vacation. She has to go back to work at the end of August at Mount St. Mary College, where she teaches nursing. In spite of Hirshel's impending spleenectomy Judi still manages to joke satirically at dinner, and Marcia and I laugh with her as always.

But I can tell that underneath her humorous exterior she's frazzled and dazed. I remember what my brave sister-in-law, Nan, and her four young children went through while my brother was battling his Hodgkin's disease. Nan had to call on reserves of strength she never knew she had. I am hoping Judi will be spared Nan's ordeal.

My friendship with the Jaffes goes back a long way. I grew up in Alexandria, Virginia; Hirshel in Brooklyn. We met in rabbinical school at the Hebrew Union College in New York City, one of the four branches of the seminary that trains rabbis for the Reform Jewish movement. Hirshel was two years behind me in school.

For a while our careers nearly coincided. He followed me into the Air Force as a chaplain. I was stationed in Japan and Korea while Hirshel served at Travis Air Force Base in California. After my discharge I became the assistant rabbi at a reform congregation in Kansas City, Missouri. Hirshel replaced me as the assistant rabbi there two years later. That's where he met Judi. She came to temple one Friday night in the summer when Hirshel was conducting Sabbath services. They were married a year later.

I moved on to a synagogue of my own in Champaign, Illinois, and Hirshel and Judi took their first pulpit in Dallas, Texas. Then I came to Manhattan to work for the American Jewish Committee, a large human relations organization. The Jaffes went to Mount Vernon, New York, and later to Newburgh.

Although we live in Manhattan and the Jaffes sixty miles upstate, we see each other often. Together we've watched our four girls, close in age, blossom into preteens. For two summers we rented cottages near each other on Martha's Vineyard, and we had some great times. Hirshel always ran circles around me with his inexhaustible brand of tennis. The Jaffes loved the Vineyard so much they found a house of their own. This was to be the summer we were at last going to take them up on their invitation to visit them in their vacation home. We were planning to drive up there later this month. Why did we put it off so long? I'm wondering. We certainly won't be making that trip now that Hirshel is ill.

Yes, friends like Hirshel and Judi are rare. Our families have shared the joys and the sorrows of life. The Jaffes mourned with us eight years ago when my brother died at the age of forty-four. And now we are agonizing over Hirshel's illness with them.

I know our relaxed friendship has meant a lot to Hirshel because it's difficult for congregational rabbis to have true friends. It's always tough to get close to your congregants. Rabbis and congregants are often inhibited in front of each other, afraid to joke or let their hair down. Congregants hire and pay the rabbi, which puts obstacles in the way of close friendships. The rabbi can never relax completely because today's congregant-friend might tomorrow be heading a faction trying to oust its spiritual leader. So we depend mainly on each other for our friends. But that's not always satisfying either because colleagues can often be backbiting and competitive.

Hirshel and I have never been professionally jealous of each other. Maybe we shouldn't get too much credit, because we are not struggling in the same arena: Hirshel is a congregational rabbi, and I am National Director of Interreligious Affairs of the AJC. So we don't vie for the same kind of recognition or for the same pulpit, and we can enjoy each other's success.

Hirshel knows he can confide in me, and he often comes to me to let off steam and ask advice. Perhaps my low-key personality complements Hirshel's hyperactive temperament. Somehow we've had the right chemistry for a real friendship throughout the years.

And friendship is so important in our tradition, adding texture to our lives even beyond the love provided by family. King David celebrates his relationship with Jonathan when he writes about his friend's death, "I grieve for you, my brother Jonathan. You were most dear to me. Your love was wonderful to me. More than the love of women." According to the Biblical Wisdom of Ben Sira, "A faithful friend is a secure shelter; whoever finds

17

one has found a treasure. A faithful friend is beyond price; his worth is more than money can buy." Hirshel Jaffe has always been my faithful friend.

After dinner we stop for doughnuts and switch Nina's and Rachel's suitcases to our station wagon. Judi gives each of them kisses. The girls seem sad to leave their mother but promise to try to have a good time.

"You can swim in the pools and lakes, play tennis and softball, ride bikes, or just hang out," Marcia tells them during the long drive back to our small vacation house, where we are spending the month of August. "You can take a ride with us in a few days when we take Jennifer up to her theater camp in the Catskills. There's so much to do, and the weather's been beautiful. You'll have a good time."

"Can I ride horses there?" Nina asks.

"I'll find out where you can rent one," Marcia promises. "We could all go. That would be fun."

The Jaffe girls say little on the long ride. Nina is carsick on the hilly, curvy mountain roads. Rachel sleeps most of the way there. Marcia and Eve and Jennifer are uncharacteristically quiet too.

In the silence I worry about Hirshel. I wonder what the prognosis is for this rare disease. I know he's nervous about the surgery tomorrow even though he put up a brave front.

I tried to do the same because I didn't want to show how worried I am. I don't want to seem anxious when I talk to him, yet I don't want to be too casual—I want him to know I'm concerned. It's really hard to strike the right balance and know what to say.

It's good that he has such a positive attitude. But that's no surprise—it's typical of Hirshel. He's always been an activist, confident he can improve the world.

18

He marched for civil rights in the 1960s, has worked for racial and religious harmony in Newburgh, even ran with a torch through the streets of New York to help free Soviet Jews. And when the Americans at our embassy in Iran were taken hostage in 1979, Hirshel went to Teheran a few months later with a group of concerned clergy and lay people. He actually met with some of the hostages to embrace them and reassure them they weren't forgotten.

The only rabbi in the group, Hirshel heard the Islamic militants spew shrill anti-Israel and anti-Jewish slogans. On the very day he went to see the hostages, the Iranians accused Hirshel of receiving "secret messages" from one of the captives. They separated him from the other Americans in the delegation and searched him. But Hirshel never lost his composure. It must have annoyed the militants when he jogged every morning around the hotel's courtyard, circling it hundreds of times during his eleven-day stay!

When Hirshel came back to the United States, he visited the hostages' families and brought them letters and welcome news from their loved ones. He organized a yellow ribbon campaign and wore a silver bracelet for one of the hostages until he was freed. Hirshel and Judi were in the White House when President Reagan officially welcomed the hostages after their release, and he's still in touch with some of them.

Hirshel is bringing this same optimism to the battle against his disease. I remember the words he spoke to me today: "I dread surgery, but I have to have it. We'll lick this! We'll use every medical technique we have. Do I have any choice?"

The truth is Hirshel does have a choice. He can simply refuse to take any action against his leukemia, even "routine" surgery like a spleenectomy. He can put his fate solely in the hands of God. That represents one religious position—trust God entirely for He is the Divine Healer, the Heavenly Physician. Intervening medically obstructs His will. Throughout history some religious groups have taught that illness, pain, and death are caused by human sinfulness. God brings suffering on us as part of a divine plan. Therefore, human beings must passively accept God's just, if apparently cruel, decisions.

But Judaism largely rejects these notions because it attaches so much importance to human life. Ours is a life-affirming religion. When Jews make a toast, they say the words *L'Hayim*, which mean "To life." The Book of Deuteronomy presents us with a clear choice. We are offered "The blessing and the curse, life or death," and we are commanded to "choose life." On Yom Kippur, the Day of Atonement, the most solemn day of our year, Jews recite the prayer, "Do not cast us away in our old age, when our strength fails us. Do not abandon us!"

According to Judaism *every* life is sacred, so everything possible must be done to save even a single soul. The many religious commandments constituting the fabric of our old and time-tested faith can be violated if a life is in danger or if there is even the risk of danger. An observant Jew who is ill may eat on Yom Kippur, the day of fasting. Physicians may perform emergency surgery on the Sabbath. All the religious commandments, except those forbidding murder, incest, or idolatry, can be waived to save a life. As one Talmudic scholar explains, "We should disregard one Sabbath for the sake of saving the life of a person so that a person may be able to observe many Sabbaths."

The rabbis tell us God cares so much for each individual life that He suffers as much as humans do when He loses one of his creatures. When even one person dies,

God's sanctity is diminished. According to Orthodox scholar Rabbi Maurice Lamm, when we say the Kaddish, the prayer for the dead, we are also comforting God because we are saying, "Your kingdom has suffered a loss; may your kingdom reign forever."

Because of the value placed on every human life, the Jewish tradition is activist and interventionist when there is human illness. It commands us to seek medical help to restore our health. This teaching created a revolution in human ethics and behavior because it demands that people participate in their own fates. So my friend must fight his disease, and he has the right to demand the same activism from his doctors and nurses.

Although Hirshel spoke impulsively, his decision to combat his leukemia is largely the result of nearly 3500 years of intense and positive interaction between Judaism and medicine. Since Biblical times there has been a long and unbroken tradition of commitment to medical treatment. Jewish scholars root the mandate to intervene medically in three Biblical verses: Exodus 21:19, "Heal, you shall surely heal"; Deuteronomy 22:2, "You shall restore it [your neighbor's ox or sheep] to your brother"; and Leviticus 19:16, "You shall not stand idly by the blood of your neighbor."

Biblical commentators note that the verb "to heal" is used twice in the Exodus verse in order to emphasize its importance. This clearly means, the scholars reason, that healing the sick is very worthwhile, is divinely ordained, and is profoundly important to God.

Moses Maimonides, the great rabbi and physician of the Middle Ages, emphasized the verse from Deuteronomy, "You shall restore it to your brother." For Maimonides, "to restore" meant not only the return of tangible physical property to a person, but also the return of physical and psychic well-being.

21

The verse from Leviticus, "You shall not stand idly by the blood of your neighbor," urges us to become active when confronted with the injured and diseased. Healing is a religious duty that falls under the Biblical commandment to save lives.

These three verses are extremely important. Because Jewish life and values are rooted in the Bible, scholars thoroughly mine every word of every sentence of the holy scriptures for meaning. By studying and interpreting these three Biblical passages, scholars developed a complex, sophisticated, and, above all, realistic system of beliefs and laws to deal with patients, physicians, drugs, illness, death, and dying.

Later scholars taught that physicians are "emmisaries of God." According to Maimonides, only a soul in a healthy body can seek out God. A physician must always try to restore a patient's health, not only for the patient's sake but so he can resume a good relationship with God.

The Physician's Prayer, attributed to Maimonides, which doctors are supposed to recite daily, emphasizes that physicians are mandated by God to heal:

> Almighty God, Thou has created the human body with infinite wisdom.
>
> Thou has blest Thine earth, Thy rivers and Thy mountains with healing substances; they enable Thy creatures to alleviate their sufferings and to heal their illnesses.
>
> Thou hast endowed man with the wisdom to relieve the suffering of his brother, to recognize his disorders, to extract the healing substances, to discover their powers and to prepare and to apply them to suit every ill.
>
> In Thine Eternal Providence Thou hast chosen me to watch over the life and health of thy creatures.

The post-Biblical writer Ben Sirah also celebrates the connection between God and the medical healer:

> Honor the doctor for his services, for the Lord created him.
> His skill comes from the Most High, and he is rewarded by kings.
> The doctor's knowledge gives him high standing and wins him the admiration of the great.
> The Lord has created medicines from the earth, and a sensible man will not disparage them. . . .
> The Lord has imparted knowledge to men, that by their use of His marvels He may win praise; by using them the doctor relieves pain and from them the pharmacist makes up his mixture.
> There is no end to the works of the Lord, who spreads health over the whole world.

However, the rabbis said, physicians must try not to fall short of their God-given task. They expected the physicians to be as proficient as possible. In the sixteenth century Rabbi Joseph Caro compared a physician who isn't an expert to a murderer.

Throughout the centuries a large body of literature has grown up in the Jewish tradition containing specific laws and regulations relating to medical practices, and this process is ongoing. Today rabbis and other scholars still heatedly debate such important contemporary bio-ethical issues as organ transplants, abortion, autopsies, the definition of death, artificial insemination, passive and active euthanasia, when to stop giving medical treatment, and medical triage—choosing who shall receive medical treatment and who shall not when choices must be made. Such discussions are not merely intellectual exercises, for the body of Jewish tradition is designed to give concrete, specific guidance to Jews in all matters of everyday life, including illness and death.

But isn't a physician interfering with God's will by trying to cure illness that is caused by God? Won't God cure people if He wants them healed? The Jewish scholars say while God ultimately controls who lives and who dies, the physician must still do everything possible to heal the sick. God creates the human body and causes illness, but we must use our intelligence to take care of it.

There is a rabbinic story in which two rabbis and a third friend walking together meet a fourth man, who is ill. After the rabbis recommend a certain medicine to the sick man, the friend protests that only God can heal. One rabbi asks the friend what his occupation is; he says he is a farmer. When the rabbi asks him if he tills the soil, he replies, "Of course, otherwise nothing would grow." The rabbi says, "Your vineyards and fields are created by God, but they can't flourish without your care. So too a human body needs care in order to survive and flourish."

Because our religion tells us we must save lives and take an active role in our medical fate, there has always been a close relationship between Judaism and doctors. The early rabbis studied the Torah and its commentaries all their lives, but they weren't paid for it, so they had other jobs; many were also physicians. Rabbi-physicians were commonplace, especially in Talmudic times (second century B.C.E. to sixth century C.E.).

Jews were required to seek out the most up-to-date, recognized medical care available. Maimonides warns us "not to live in a city that has no physician." A fourteenth-century rabbi taught, "Nowadays one must not rely on miracles, and the ill person is duty bound to call a physician in order to be healed. To claim greater merit than the many righteous people of the past who were healed by doctors is almost as sinful as a reliance on miracles. One should adopt the ways of men and be healed by a physician."

The Jewish tradition urges us to practice preventive medicine as well. Of the 613 religious commandments a Jew is expected to observe, 213, more than one third of the total, are medical in nature. They regulate almost every aspect of daily life. These laws deal with personal and community hygiene, including the washing of the body, rules of sexual cleanliness, care of the skin, dietary laws, isolation and quarantine, the proper care of garments and cooking utensils, and public health practices for cities and villages.

The Talmud also has many specific references to preventive medicine. Mar Samuel, perhaps the greatest medical practitioner mentioned in the Talmud and the king of Persia's personal physician, taught that the "washing of hands and feet in the morning and evening are more effective than any remedy." This emphasis on preventive medicine and awareness of the relationship between personal hygiene and health, dating back to Biblical times, was far advanced for its time.

But the rabbis never forget the role faith and prayer also play in healing the body. These two equal forces—active medical procedures and active personal and communal prayers—are both gifts from God, and both are required for successful treatment. The rabbis constantly insist on using both physicians and prayers; each one is necessary, but if used alone, insufficient.

August 3, 1982

It's nine o'clock now. The hospital switchboard is closed. No more telephone calls from my friends and family or congregants. No more visitors. My roommate is asleep.

I'm alone with my thoughts.

I never knew how scary hospitals are at night. The glare from the hallway invades your room. It's never really quiet. Someone is always walking up and down the corridor, and the phone rings at the nurses' station. I'm sure I won't sleep at all tonight.

The doctors and the anesthesiologist came in today to explain tomorrow's procedures. They said this operation is routine, nothing to worry about. But is any surgery really "routine"? Judi has told me some horror stories. And with my leukemia, bleeding could be a problem.

What happens if my blood counts don't bounce back after they take out my spleen, and my disease doesn't go into remission? What other kinds of treatment will work? What can they do for me then? I wonder if the doctors even know.

How long will I live? That day with Judi in the hematologist's office when I asked him how long people live with this disease, he said, "Well, six months, two years, ten years . . ." I guess they just don't know.

Jim really pushed me this afternoon and started me thinking. He asked me if I felt God is punishing me and if I'm angry at God. Now that I'm alone and the night is so long and I am just lying here waiting for tomorrow, I am beginning to wonder why this is happening to me. Why is this happening to me? Do I deserve this? Have I done something wrong or been a bad person? Am I being punished?

Why should someone like me who's trying to "do God's work," a rabbi trying to preserve Judaism and help people lead better Jewish lives, be afflicted? Is this the "reward" I get? This illness will interfere with my goals. Doesn't God want me to succeed? Then why would He put such a difficult stumbling block in my way? It doesn't make sense.

But wait a minute. Is God really involved in this at all? Is He concerned with the life of one little person, even one dedicated to serving Him? Could God have prevented this disease?

Can He cure me? If God does have the power, do I have enough faith to believe He will help me?

That internist I went to, a Muslim, first brought up the question of faith. The last thing he said to me was, "Well, Rabbi Jaffe, we must have faith." That's when I knew I was really in trouble. There's something very scary about those words. But he meant them sincerely. I wonder if that doctor believes in God more than I do. Do I really believe in God? What kind of God do I believe in? Will He help me?

I just listened to a Willie Nelson tape through my earphones. His music always makes me feel good, but tonight the words really got to me. It was almost like he was singing them just for me, and I couldn't help thinking about my past and my future as I listened to the music. He sang, "Maybe I didn't love you quite as often as I could have, maybe I didn't treat you quite as good as I should have." That made me think about Judi and the kids. Have I loved them enough? Have I taken care of them? Why didn't I get more life insurance? I certainly can't get any more coverage now.

That song made me feel I don't want to be alone now; I need to be connected to other people—Judi, the children, all my friends. And my parents. I sure wish they were here with me now, but I know it's hard for them to cope with my illness, and they're upset. My dad probably just can't believe or doesn't want to believe I am seriously ill. My folks told my uncle that I have anemia. I said, "Mom, it's leukemia, don't hide it. I want it out in the open."

I know I shouldn't be impatient with my parents. I've always been their little pride and joy. They're probably still thinking that their bright, shiny little Hirshel, their firstborn, will pull off another great miracle, that I'll run another marathon for them. . . .

Maybe I'll never finish another marathon or run as far or as fast, but I know I'll run again. I guess that's what I think about most, my running. The first question I asked the

27

hematologist when he told us I had leukemia was, "Will I ever run again?" I felt so relieved when he said, "Hirshel, we'll have you running again by Rosh Hashana." But that's only seven weeks away. I hope I'll be well enough by then.

We get back to our house in the Poconos about 10 P.M. I carry Nina's and Rachel's suitcases into the house, and Marcia makes up their beds.

We all fall into bed exhausted.

Hirshel's surgery is scheduled for 8 A.M. tomorrow.

There is nothing to do now but wait.

3

~~~

J udi telephones us about dinnertime. Hirshel has come through the surgery well, but he's still in the intensive care unit.

"They're just being cautious," she assures us. "They want to keep an eye on him. The surgery wasn't so routine. When they got his spleen out, they found it was as big as a grapefruit. I think they got it out just in time. It would have ruptured soon. But his blood counts bounced back up immediately. They told Hirshel as soon as he came out of the anesthesia, and that really lifted his spirits. So the surgery was a success. The leukemia is arrested. He should be getting his energy back soon."

When we telephone Hirshel a few days later, we're relieved to find he's out of intensive care and back in his room, but we're surprised his voice is so weak.

"There's so much pain, Jim . . . I didn't realize it would be this bad. I just wasn't prepared for this. . . . Surgery was so scary, Jim. When I was in the ICU, a horrifying thing happened. I was just waking up from the anesthesia, I was so disoriented, and I heard this loud alarm going off. I panicked and screamed for help. The alarm was from the bed next to mine. . . . They gave me breakfast the day after the operation, but I started having stomach pains, and now they're feeding me through an

IV tube. But my blood count went from 20,000 to 200,000 platelets. So that's great. . . . Good-bye."

Hirshel hangs up before I can say another word.

We telephone him every night about eight-thirty after all his visitors are gone and we know he will be facing the loneliness of a long hospital night. But he isn't getting stronger. A week after the surgery Hirshel is still in a lot of pain and feeling miserable. Marcia and I are beginning to fear something's going wrong.

"They want me to get up and walk around," Hirshel tells me, "but when I try to walk through the halls, pushing my IV monitor, I lurch and double up with cramps and hiccoughing. I don't understand what's happening. The nurses say you have to expect these side effects. Sometimes you get a partial paralysis of the bowels following anesthesia, and maybe mine is just lasting a little longer than usual. I just know I'm not recovering normally. You know how impatient I am. I wanted to get out of here in a few days like the doctors promised and be up on the Vineyard.

"I still can't eat or drink anything. But the worst thing is it's so hard to move because of these IVs in my arms. . . . I feel so confined. When you came to visit, you told me I looked like a jogger in jail. Well, now I do feel like a prisoner hooked up to all these scary, beeping monitors. If my Greenhaven Prison inmates could see me now . . . Their chaplain who always zipped in and out the front gate to freedom is now a prisoner just like them."

A few nights later on the phone Hirshel complains the physicians seem to blame him for not recovering. "They act like I'm not trying hard enough. They keep saying if I move around more my intestines will start to work. They're chiding me for not getting out of bed more. But,

Jim, I don't feel like getting up. I'm too weak and it hurts too much. And I'm not getting enough calories just with the IV. I'm losing weight every day. I always wanted to be thin, but this is ridiculous."

"What do the doctors say?" Marcia, on the extension telephone, asks.

"Well, my surgeon is on vacation. But I hope he gets back soon because the other doctors don't seem to want to act without him. Sometimes they don't take my complaints seriously, so I get pushy. Then they lecture me and make me feel like I'm just a big baby. Or they pacify me by saying they'd be just as upset as I am. But I know it's not my fault that I'm not getting better. I know my body's not responding, and I'm getting weaker instead of stronger. Look, I can't talk anymore. I'm hanging up now. . . ."

"Is the pain getting any better?" I ask Hirshel the next time we phone him.

"No. They give me shots for it, thank God. I never thought I'd be using strong painkillers. You know me, Jim, I never took anything, hardly even aspirin. I always thought it was a sign of weakness to take drugs. I even have to take sleeping pills now because my body won't relax and I can't sleep. I feel like I'm almost getting addicted to these Demerol shots. I barely took any medication before, and now all of a sudden I feel like I'm becoming a junkie.

"But I take them. Have to. It hurts too much, and they relieve me. But in a way they make things worse, because they make me so woozy, and Judi says they're slowing down my intestines. It's a vicious cycle. And I don't like being so dependent on them. It's partly a matter of pride. Some nurses make subtle little remarks about how many painkillers I'm taking. Others say, 'Don't be such a hero, go ahead and take them.' But I feel like I'm fighting a battle with myself because I'm going against my instinct, which is to be healthy and natural. I've always stayed away from medications and been so health-conscious and athletic because I think keeping your body pure celebrates and praises God."

Hirshel's observation reminds me of a long and beautiful passage in the *Zohar,* a book of religious mysticism written primarily in the thirteenth century, where the Jewish mystics say the human body is a reflection of the entire miraculous universe.

In other ancient religions and philosophies the body and soul represented conflicting cosmic forces of good and evil. The human body, physical existence, interfered with pure spiritual fulfillment, so life on this earth was considered a barrier to happiness and eternal life. But for Judaism body and soul are not at odds. They depend on each other. Both are expressions of the holy. Human life is an important part of God's creation and is supremely valuable.

God's interest in the life and bodies of all His creatures is a fundamental concept of Jewish law. We're supposed to enjoy life. The rabbis always urged us to be moderate in eating, drinking, and sexual activity, but we're not supposed to be ascetic. And we shouldn't do anything to hurt our bodies.

Hirshel's desire to keep his system free of drugs also conforms to Jewish teachings. A twelfth-century rabbi is astonishingly modern when he advises, "Do not take drugs because they demand periodic doses and your heart will crave them. You will also lose money. Even for medicinal purposes do not take drugs if you can find a different medicine that will help."

Yet, although the rabbis generally discouraged using drugs, they condoned taking painkillers if needed. If pain keeps you from functioning and relating to your family or to God, you must try to ease it, and you may even violate the Sabbath to do so. You may give any drugs to the terminally ill to make their last days more comfortable and pain-free, even if they are experimental medications and even if they actually shorten the patient's life.

As the days go by, Marcia and I get more and more worried about Hirshel. We try to hide our fears from the Jaffe girls, but they can sense something's wrong, and they're very anxious about their father too. None of us is enjoying our Pocono mountain "paradise" anymore.

To our dismay, the next time we phone Hirshel he seems weaker and has frequent hiccoughs.

"I have these terrible abdominal pains," he whispers, "and my stomach is distended. Something is blocking my stomach and preventing me from eating. They can't give me enough calories through my IV. Jim, my body is so weak it has become chemically imbalanced. . . . And now I have this horrible tube they put through my nose into my stomach to relieve the pains and bloating and measure my stomach contents."

"Can't they do anything about the blockage?"

"They don't seem to know what to do. They're still hesitating and hoping I'll come around. But it's been fourteen days now, and I'm going crazy in here. I think they're scared to do anything till the surgeon gets back from his vacation in a few days. I know they're stalling —they can't even look me straight in the eye. But I'm on to them. I yelled at one of the doctors, I called him a shit-head. Jim, I never dreamed I'd have these complications.

I thought I'd be in this hospital for a short time and then I'd be on my way to the Vineyard. God, was I ever naïve. I can see that now. The summer is slipping by. I feel trapped in here. I feel like a hostage—a hostage to this hospital and to all these machines.

"And you know, we always think physicians are gods. Now I'm finding out they're only human like everybody else. It makes me nervous to see the anxiety in my doctors' eyes and hear them talking among themselves. Sometimes they all stand at the foot of my bed and talk about me like I'm not even here, like I'm just a little kid that can't understand what they're saying. It makes you feel invisible.

"The nurses are only human too. The hospital is frantic, and they run all over. It's hard to know which one is yours. Some of them have no idea why I had my spleen out. They don't connect it with leukemia, so they don't realize why I'm here. It's hard for me to rely on nurses for everything and be so dependent. I've always taken charge of my own life, and now I have to ring the buzzer and wait for them to come. Sometimes it seems like forever.

"And they rarely have time to talk to you. There is one nice social worker who seems to understand me. She listens sympathetically and asks me where my head is at. It's good therapy to talk to someone. I wish more people were here to talk to Hirshel the person, not just to Hirshel the patient."

I can see now how important it is for Marcia and me to keep telephoning Hirshel every night, even though it's painful for us to talk to him while he's in such bad shape. He needs to have somebody he can complain to, somebody to chat with and to make him relax.

"You know, people have always complained that their

physicians are sometimes insensitive," I assure Hirshel. "There's a lot in the Talmud about good doctor-patient relationships. The rabbis urged doctors to treat the whole person, not just the ailment."

"Like the new holistic medicine Judi keeps talking about."

"It isn't so new, Hirshel. Some of those ideas are in the Talmud. Look, you need your sleep. We'll phone you again tomorrow. Keep on fighting—you'll start to feel better soon, I know it."

Hirshel's doctors ought to be reciting the Physician's Prayer, I think after I hang up the telephone. The prayer reminds them of their profession's high moral and ethical standards and of how crucial it is to treat the patient with humanity—to heal and consider the whole person, not just the specific illness. "Inspire me with love for my art and for Thy creatures," the physician implores God.

> Do not allow thirst for profit, ambition for renown and admiration, to interfere with my profession, for these are the enemies of truth and of love for mankind and they can lead astray in the great task of attending to the welfare of Thy creatures. Preserve the strength of my body and of my soul that they ever be ready to cheerfully help and support rich and poor, good and bad, enemy as well as friend. *In the sufferer let me see only the human being.* (Italics added.)

Rabbinic scholars urged physicians to have a good bedside manner. Doctors should be frank with patients about their medical condition, but should break bad news gently. The rabbis relate how Moses told his brother, Aaron, of Aaron's approaching death as an example of how to handle this issue sensitively. According to the legend, Moses sat down with Aaron and read the story of the creation of the world, but when they reached the description of the creation of Adam, Moses said, "I don't know if I can call the creation of man good when man must die." Aaron said, "We must resign ourselves to the will of God." Moses took advantage of this opening to tell his brother he would soon die.

Apparently even in Talmudic times many were cynical about physicians. One fifteenth-century Biblical scholar comments, "The knavish doctor is the colleague of the angel of death." Another says, "The best of physicians belongs in hell!" Jedadiah ben Abraham Bedersi, a fourteenth-century French Jewish poet and philosopher, writes:

> When you need a physician, you esteem him a god;
> When he has brought you out of danger, you consider
>   him a king.
> When you have been cured, he becomes human like
>   yourself;
> When he sends you the bill, you think him a devil.

The rabbis even discussed appropriate doctors' fees. Physicians were never to charge the poor or to deny treatment to those who cannot pay. Doctors were not supposed to receive fees for their services—they were only to be paid for the interruption of their time. However, most doctors did get paid, and, in fact, the Talmud advises, "A doctor who charges nothing is worth nothing!" An Egyptian physician writes, "The more you demand for your service, the greater will it appear in the eyes of the people. Your art will be looked down upon by people you treat for nothing."

These passages show us that people haven't changed. As I agonize with Hirshel now, I realize how astoundingly fresh and up-to-date our nearly 3500-year-old religion is.

I've been in the hospital for seventeen days, and I can't understand why my parents aren't here with me yet. I'm really sick. I need them.

My brother Ronnie is coming from California in a few days. My brother Bob doesn't live far from here, and he called to say he's coming. He just sent me another Willie Nelson tape. My parents call me from Martha's Vineyard every day, sometimes twice a day. They ask a million questions, but if I tell them anything too bleak or pessimistic they can't stand to hear it. So it's hard for me to let my true feelings out. They've gotten so emotional they're nearly paralyzed into inaction.

Maybe my parents are doing all they can. They keep saying how hard it is for them to come. My mother says my dad can't handle coming here. He's not eating because he's so worried about me and he's losing weight. She doesn't want to leave him and come here by herself. They say they anguish over me every minute.

They've always relied on me for strength. Maybe it's because I'm a rabbi. They've leaned on me and come to me for comfort and advice when there was trouble in the family. But now they can see I am the one who needs to be comforted by them, and I think that's hard for them to deal with. It's hard for me too, because I have never had to turn to other people before. Like Ronnie, he's always been my "little brother," and I always worried about him. Now our roles are reversed. And Robert has depended on me in the past. But now I can't be his pillar anymore. At least not for a while.

At night after my visitors leave and my telephone calls stop and I'm alone in here, I can't sleep even with the shots they give me. So I watch all-night cable news on the little TV set above my bed.

I see Arabs and Jews fighting in Lebanon. There are other wars in the world, and it all seems so hopeless to me now. I'm getting so cynical about everything. I say to myself, "If that's what life is all about, then nothing is ever going to be healed. I'm not ever going to be healed . . . the world isn't ever going to be healed." I keep watching television and thinking about myself, about my own destructibility.

And day by day I am sadly realizing we'll never have our vacation on Martha's Vineyard.

I had already lashed our bicycles to the roof of our jeep for the trip to the Vineyard when the internist finally decided something was seriously wrong with my blood and told me not to go away. So I took the bikes down and canceled the ferry reservations. That was symbolic. I was terribly disappointed. My next-door neighbor was really startled when he saw me unloading the jeep because he knew how much I wanted to get up to our house, and he's never seen me change my plans.

Yesterday I looked out of my hospital window and saw a little airplane flying low. I thought, if only I could get on that plane I'd be free, I'd fly over to Martha's Vineyard and be jogging on the beach with Rachel and Nina and driving our jeep over the sand dunes.

The license plate on our Golden Eagle Jeep says **Nesher**, the Hebrew word for "eagle." There's a passage in Isaiah having to do with eagles: "You shall be lifted. Those who wait on the Lord shall renew their strength; they shall mount up with wings like eagles. They shall run and not be weary. They shall walk and not be faint." Maybe that should be my motto now.

I used to quote those words when people asked me why I was so addicted to running. Some think that Biblical passage refers to immortality. I guess that's when I still thought running would make me live forever. I once read an article by a

Christian minister on why people run. He says we're trying to
run away from death.

Well, I can't "mount up with wings like eagles" now. I can't
fly away on that airplane. I can't even disconnect my tubes
and just walk away.

Will I ever be free?

4

Rachel and Nina Jaffe have stopped going to the beaches and pools. They don't want to do anything even though the weather is still almost perfect. Nina doesn't even want to ride horses, she's so upset about her father's condition.

Finally I tell Hirshel on the telephone, "I think your kids have had it. They want to go home. We'll take them to your hospital and meet Judi there."

"Jim, I'm finally hearing the truth. One physician told me I might need a second operation to correct the blockage."

"Oh, no!"

"Yes. But they can't guarantee it's going to be successful. If they operate again and it doesn't work, then how will I ever get out of here? Do you know what my chances are of withstanding more surgery? I don't know if I can pull through—I'm so weak now. I could have more bleeding because of my leukemia. During the spleenectomy they had to give me lots of extra blood because mine wasn't clotting. But, Jim, they have to do something. I can't go on like this anymore. My surgeon comes back from his vacation tomorrow, and he's going to be very upset to see me like this. It's probably too late for him to do anything now."

"Hirshel, don't say that! It's not like you to talk like that!"

"I know, Jim. I can feel myself slipping. I have these dark forebodings. I'm so afraid, Jim, it's hard for me to talk about this, but I know I can tell you, because you'll understand. I'm afraid I'm going to die. . . . For the first time in my life I'm facing death. And I feel so helpless, Jim. I don't have my old willpower. I'm almost too resigned, too tranquil, and I know that's dangerous. It's like I'm fading. I'm beginning to wonder why I should keep fighting if I don't have a chance. Is life worth this struggle?"

"Of course it is. Look at all you have to live for. Hirshel—you can't give up now."

I am thinking to myself, "It's easy for you, Jim, to say, 'Don't give up hope.' It's not *you* lying in that hospital bed day after day, staring death in the face."

"I know everybody's telling me I can't give up, that I have to fight, and I'm trying to," Hirshel pleads, "but I'm so afraid it's all for nothing, that I'm just going to die. I can't keep pretending I'm a hero when I don't feel like one anymore. It's hard to keep fighting when my doctors hesitate, and they're running out of places to put my IV, and my veins are collapsing. Everything is going wrong. I think it's too late, Jim. There's nothing they can do for me now."

"Hirshel, don't be so passive! You can't just give up. The Torah says, 'choose life,' remember?" I know I must sound like an obnoxious cheerleader to Hirshel, and he hardly needs lessons in Judaism. But I'm trying everything I can to shake my friend out of his despair.

"I'm just not sure it's my choice anymore, Jim."

"Don't give up, Hirshel," I beg him again. "You're going to pull through this, I know."

42

"I wish I could be so sure. Jim . . . thanks for being such a good friend," Hirshel whispers as he hangs up.

"What the hell is going on in that hospital?!" Marcia shouts from the bedroom, where she has been listening to our conversation on the extension phone. We decide to call a mutual friend of ours and the Jaffes' who is on the staff of Hirshel's hospital.

"What's happening with Hirshel?" I scream into the phone.

"Now, Jim, calm down," our friend advises. "It isn't as bad as Hirshel thinks. He's had some complications, but he'll recover. Hirshel is just very depressed right now. This is awfully hard for him to handle, and he has good reason to be upset. But he's in more danger from his depression than from the stomach problem. If he doesn't pull out of his panic and gloom, his physical condition could get even worse, and then he really could die. He's losing hope and giving up his fight, and that's dangerous."

"Hirshel feels he's losing control over his own life," Marcia observes after we say good-bye to our friend. "And I'm sure all those tubes and IVs are robbing him of his dignity."

"Marcia, even the Talmudic rabbis recognized that patients often feel powerless and cut off from making important decisions. So they urged visitors to take concrete steps to help them feel important. They suggested specific activities to give patients, even the hopelessly ill, a feeling of power and control over their lives when they are feeling so vulnerable.

"Visitors should urge patients to write down last-minute advice to their children about how to live a good life, especially when they didn't have much money or property to leave them. The rabbis said we should encourage patients to record their life stories so their families can read them, and make sure they keep donating to charity so they'll feel they're still an important part of society."

The delicate and complex interrelationship between the mind and the body in causing and curing serious illness has been recognized for centuries, my wife, who used to teach philosophy and religion, points out to me. The Greek physician Hippocrates recognized the importance of the patient's role in overcoming illness and the great difference positive feelings between patient and physician can make. "Some patients," the ancient Greek physician wrote, "though conscious that their condition is perilous, recover their health simply with their contentment with the goodness of the physician."

A passage in the Biblical Wisdom of Ben Sira advises, "Do not give yourself over to sorrow or distress yourself deliberately. A merry heart keeps a man alive, and joy lengthens his space of days. . . . Envy and anger shorten a man's life, and anxiety brings premature old age."

Maimonides wrote in the twelfth century, "Emotional experiences cause marked changes in the body which are clear and visible to all . . . the physician should do nothing before he improves the soul by removing the extreme emotions. In order to strengthen the vital powers," he advises, "one should employ musical instruments and tell patients gay stories which will make the heart swell and narratives that will distract the mind and cause them and their friends to laugh. One should select as attendants and caretakers those who can cheer up the patient. . . ." Maimonides' axiom, "A healthy soul in a healthy body," presaged modern insights about how important a positive state of mind is in overcoming illness.

I am passionately hoping that when Marcia and I visit Hirshel tomorrow we will help him regain his "healthy

44

soul." I pray that our visit will rally Hirshel to fight for his life.

Jewish scholars always realized how much influence bedside visitors can have on a patient's state of mind and how important a patient's positive psychological outlook can be for his physical recovery. Nearly two thousand years ago the great Rabbi Akiba warned that one who does not visit the sick is like one who sheds blood, because he causes further illness and even death. Another Talmudic scholar taught, "He who visits the sick causes him to recover, and he who does not visit the sick causes him to die." These ancient beliefs, based on incredibly modern insights, have been confirmed by modern scientists.

Visiting the sick, *Bikur Holim* in Hebrew, is a sacred obligation for *every* Jew, an important religious duty—a *Mitzvah*—not merely a voluntary or a social activity. *Bikur Holim,* one of the most important requirements of our religion, is so powerful that Jewish tradition claims God Himself visited Abraham following the patriarch's circumcision!

Long before socialized medicine and modern health insurance, the European Jewish communities organized *Bikur Holim* associations that provided physicians, druggists, hospital attendants, and midwives. These publicly supported societies offered every Jew free complete medical coverage from birth to death. They cared for the poor in hospitals founded by the Jewish community. Volunteer societies of women served as nurses, offered prayers, sewed shrouds, and ritually prepared dead women for burial. No sick person, rich or poor, was to be left alone without medical care or visitors.

The Jewish tradition sets out strict rules regarding the visits themselves. First offer material assistance to the patient. Then recite special, personal prayers for the ill during every visit. Some of the earliest recorded prayers in Judaism are prayers for the sick.

Today we sometimes misunderstand and minimize the meaning of prayers for the ill because we often think praying is a sign of weakness or superstition. The Jewish concept of prayer is not just that we ask God for something, in this case to heal the patient. The Hebrew word for prayer means to "examine or search one's self or soul." The Talmud cautions us to pray "without seeking fulfillment." We are being presumptuous if we think God must answer our prayers.

So visitors' prayers for the ill are not mechanistic incantations that will automatically cure the patient. The main purpose of prayer is to overcome despair and depression and help stir patients and their families to act positively. We must understand prayer as a healing force in a broad therapeutic sense. In Judaism prayers not only "go up" to God; they must "go out" to other people and "go in" to ourselves as well. Prayers make us introspective and link us with the ill person who desperately needs our affection and support.

Prayer can be a kind of psychotherapy, both for the patient and for the healthy visitor, benefiting not only the patient but also the visitor who prays. According to the Talmud, whoever prays for the ill has his own prayers answered first. So the praying visitor fulfills his own needs and improves his own psychological condition while at the same time helping the patient.

The Jewish tradition encourages visitors to come often, even on the Sabbath. Don't come too early or too late or stay too long and fatigue the patient. Be cheerful. Leave every patient with hope. Be a good listener and talk specifically about the illness—don't try to avoid the subject. Don't be what the Talmud calls a stupid visitor —that is, one who mindlessly tells a patient something insensitive, such as "Oh, my father died of your disease."

At all times visitors must respect the patient's dignity. Jewish tradition says, for example, that you shouldn't hover over the patient's bed. Sit instead in a chair on an equal level with the patient. If you stand over the bed he has to look up, which intensifies his feeling of powerlessness. But if you sit down, the patient feels less lonely and more part of a social group and community.

Good visitors don't morally judge patients, like Job's friends who sharply questioned him and implied that he was somehow responsible for his own misfortunes. Hirshel Jaffe's visitors must calm his fears, help overcome his loneliness, and give him strength to confront his pain and anxieties.

Suddenly leaving behind and losing contact with the people you love and need when you are so vulnerable can be shattering. Visitors are concrete links to our normal lives, a sign of solidarity, forming a human bridge to the world outside the hospital.

Visitors themselves can gain from the experience a sense of their own fragility. If leukemia can strike an always healthy, young marathon runner like Hirshel Jaffe, who never smoked, always ate the right food, and exercised constantly, then who is safe? A visit to an ill friend renews our own sense of vulnerability.

And visits to the sick represent a kind of unspoken but potentially powerful board of review of the patient's medical team. Hirshel Jaffe's many visitors must be positively influencing his doctors, for they see that so many people care deeply about him. Just by being there, Hirshel's visitors form a sort of human life insurance policy for him.

～～～～

Am I going to die?

I'm thinking a lot about my life, especially since I have so much time on my hands and I can hardly move. I am lying here thinking every kind of thought, from sexual fantasies, to how selfish I've been, to things I should have done for people. I'm conscious of all the things I could have done and wish I had done. Maybe God is punishing me for not doing enough with my life. Have I wasted it, frittered away my time? Am I a failure? I've tried to be a good rabbi, but maybe I haven't measured up to the task. Maybe I've been too vain and arrogant. I hope I get another chance to prove myself.

But whatever I've done or haven't done, I certainly don't think I deserve to die. I don't want to die. I have so much work left to do. Why would God let me die before I've finished it? And I don't want to leave my wife and children. . . .

I am so lucky to have Judi. Lots of wives would have fallen apart by now. But she's still joking and bawling me out for not feeling better and badgering me and telling me not to give up, dammit. She's nagging me for my own good, and I know that her biting humor is the only way she can deal with this situation.

And I know how lucky I am to have so many wonderful friends showing such concern for me. The visitors keep me going even though sometimes it's hard for me to prepare for them. I don't know if I should take my medication before they come because I know it makes me drowsy. I feel dirty and I look awful, and sometimes I don't feel like playing the genial host. I'm used to being on top of everything and sort of above everybody because I'm a rabbi; now I'm in bad shape and vulnerable. It's degrading to have people see me like this. But the good outweighs the bad. When my visitors come it is always good.

When I get back to work, I'll make more hospital stops, and

I'll know sometimes patients feel degraded as I do now. I won't think of my visits as just part of my job. Sometimes I used to get them over with as quickly as possible. I won't do that anymore. I'll make sure the doctors are giving patients and their families all the information they need because now I know how terrifying it is to be in the dark about your condition.

I'll take more time to listen to the patient's anxieties instead of just giving my routine assurances, as I did too often. And I'll pay more attention to the family's anguish, because I can see now that the illness deeply affects the entire family. I'll make sure I give the family a lot of special counseling. I'll keep checking on the patient and the family instead of going just once or twice.

My friend Stephanie is at the hospital almost constantly. She hovers over me and caters to me and cheers me up. Her husband, Jonathan, is unofficially monitoring the way the other doctors are handling my case. Stephanie and Jonathan delayed their vacation because they're so worried about me. Ironically, they were supposed to go to Martha's Vineyard too. They even brought their son to visit me here. He is a sensitive boy, but little did I dream that this twelve-year-old child would approach my bed and nestle me in his arms as I cuddled him and that he would cry because he cared for me. I'll never forget it. It was beautiful. It gave me such comfort.

Rabbi Sy Dresner stops by to trade rabbinical stories, and my classmate Ronnie Millstein visits and phones. Alan and Paula from my congregation come to visit me, and I talk to Paula on the phone frequently. They're so good at lifting my spirits. What a lot they have to cope with! Paula had Hodgkin's disease when she was younger, and then she gave birth to a Down's syndrome child years later. We came home from the Vineyard to be with them the summer it happened. Paula really understands what I'm going through, because she battled cancer, and now she's helping me to face my illness. And Alan is so wise and supportive. He's such a decent guy.

49

Two prominent members of my congregation came to see me last night. They painstakingly spoon-fed me Jell-O, dodging the tubes in my mouth. What a considerate thing to do. I'm sure it wasn't very pleasant for them. One of them is a lawyer. Judi told me this morning that he offered to give her free legal advice if she needs it. I guess he means in case I die. Judi says rumors are going around the congregation that I'm not going to make it.

Other congregants telephone me. My president and my cantor too. What great guys. My cantor visits me a lot here and walks me around the halls, steadying me as I push my IV pole.

I know my congregants are trying to protect me. They don't want to upset me now. Yesterday I discovered by chance that Joan, our temple bookkeeper, died. She had bone cancer. When my cantor came to the hospital, I looked at him and said, "Joan died, didn't she?" He said, "Oh, my God, Hirshel, we weren't supposed to tell you." I found out where Joan's family was in mourning and telephoned them. I want still to function as a rabbi. I don't want to be cut off from everybody and from my duties.

Even the inmates in Greenhaven Prison sent me a big get-well card. They all signed it, just like little kids in school. There must be twenty names on the card. Somebody opened the card for me and said, "Hey, what's this, what are all these names?" It must have taken a lot of effort to pass the card around and get those signatures and find out what hospital their chaplain is in. Prisoners hesitate to sign their names to things. It's touching to think these cynical men care about me. You wouldn't imagine they'd be concerned about another person. Usually they're only out for themselves, worried about their appeals or when their parole is coming up.

Of course, it's not just my Jewish friends who have helped me. Reverend Glen Henricksen and Father Tom Fenlon from Newburgh came to pray with me. I'm on everybody's prayer list. But will their prayers do any good? Will anyone's?

Today Rabbi Marty Freedman came to visit. Marty is so reassuring, with his deep, strong voice. And he knows a lot about medicine. He talked to my doctors to make sure they're doing the right thing.

I guess I've never realized the power of a personal blessing. It's not really a matter of theology. It's the strength of one human being praying for another, praying to God. I was vulnerable and childlike and clinging to Marty's hand. My feelings welled up inside of me, and I looked up at him, and tears came into my eyes, and he spoke to me reassuringly. I told him how much I love Judi and Rachel and Nina, and I said, "Rabbi, hold my hand and give me your blessing." He did give me his blessing, and I realized how much my bringing comfort has meant to all the people I have visited these past twenty years and why people are showing me such love and concern now.

After Marty left, I remembered a story we learned in rabbinical school illustrating how we need the prayers and support of others to recover. The great Talmudic sage Rabbi Yohanan became ill and a colleague visited him. When the friend was about to leave, Rabbi Yohanan said, "Give me your hand." The visitor held his hand. The Talmud says that Yohanan was at that moment cured because, like the prisoner who cannot free himself from prison, so, too, the patient cannot free himself from illness without outside help.

Like Rabbi Yohanan, I had asked a colleague to hold my hand and pray for my recovery, to help me break free from the spiritual prison of my illness and the physical prison of my hospital room.

Maybe this is where God comes into all this: He is present in the love and concern of people for each other. He tries to help you learn to cope with your destiny and to accept it. God is in the power of love, the power of prayer, the power of human faith, the power of a blessing like Marty's.

It means so much to know everybody's cheering me on from

the sidelines as they did during the New York Marathon four years ago. I knew I'd make the whole twenty-six miles because people were with me. That's what's so wonderful about running. You feel like you're part of humanity, you feel like everybody's applauding just for you. Well, I feel everybody is cheering me on now too, but I don't know if I'm going to make it this time. . . . I really don't know. . . .

This is one race I might not finish.

5

~~~~~

Anxious and nervous, early the next morning we drive as quickly as possible to the hospital to visit Hirshel and to return the Jaffe girls to Judi. When we get there, I call up to Hirshel's room. Ronnie, his youngest brother, answers Hirshel's telephone and soon comes down to the lobby. He looks strained and worried. Ronnie stays with Rachel and Nina while Marcia and I hurry up to Hirshel's room.

We're shocked when we see our friend. He is pale and emaciated, nearly wasted away. A tube reaching down to his stomach to relieve his pains and distension hangs from his nose. The IV unit through which he is receiving an enriched feeding formula envelops his body. It is a different Hirshel Jaffe. He doesn't even try to smile when he sees us.

"Look what Ronnie did," Hirshel says as he points with his free hand to the wall above his bed. "He pinned my 'Running Rabbi' T-shirt right underneath my marathon picture. I guess that's his way of giving me a pep talk. God, I need one now . . . so good to see Ronnie."

"What's the latest, Hirshel?" I ask.

"My surgeon is due back from his vacation this morning. Maybe they'll finally do something. This is so ironic. Here I've been winning the battle with my leukemia. My blood count is better now so that isn't the problem at the moment. But I still might lose the war. The disease may not kill me, but complications from a 'routine' operation might.

"Jim, I said before I didn't think God was responsible for my illness. But now I have to wonder if God is maybe testing me. Maybe He wants to see if I have a strong enough character to handle this. Is God playing tricks on me or trying to fool me? Or maybe this is just a trick by Mother Nature. Is it all just fate?

"On Rosh Hashana we ask, 'Who will die of hunger or thirst?' That's hitting close to home with me now. Maybe God has ordained that I will die 'by hunger and by thirst' now, and there's just not a thing we can do about it. What good is all this medicine and surgery? I might as well just give up. . . ."

A pleasant-looking man in his sixties rushes into the hospital room. Hirshel manages a weak smile and introduces Marcia and me to his surgeon. We turn our backs as he raises Hirshel's hospital gown and examines his abdominal area carefully. The surgeon seems shocked to find Hirshel in this condition even though he was probably briefed by the other physicians. He is obviously extremely concerned.

"There are definitely adhesions in your stomach blocking your intestines as a result of the spleenectomy," the surgeon announces. "That's why you can't digest your food. I'm operating this morning. Now! The nurses will come in to prep you right away." He removes Hirshel's tubes and puts his hand on Hirshel's shoulder. "You'll make it, Rabbi. I have faith that you'll make it."

Marcia wanders over to the window and stares outside. I sit down in the chair next to Hirshel's bed and take my friend's hand in mine. I am surprised that his grip is still so strong.

"This might be it, Jim. I don't know if I'm going to

pull through this. . . . Thanks for being such a good friend. Be sure to say thanks to everyone for me . . . for everything they have done. Thank Marty Freedman and all my other friends. . . ."

As Hirshel holds my hand and looks at me, I see the fear in his eyes, his sophisticated psychological defenses blown away. I listen helplessly as my friend utters this muted cry of anguish from his hospital bed. It is the oldest cry in the world and unites Hirshel with every other human being who has ever lived, become ill, and faced death. It is a wild explosion of questions, anger, resentments, and cries from the heart. Why me? Why Hirshel Jaffe? Why in the prime of my life?

"Jim, what would the great Professor Atlas say to me now if he were alive?" Hirshel asks, reminding me of our long-ago teacher. "Would he have the answers for me? Could he tell me why I'm suffering like this? Is there a reason? Does it mean anything? Why is God putting me through this?"

"Hirshel, this is no time for a heavy discussion. You're not up to it and neither am I. First things first. Let's get your body working and get you out of here. Then we can talk. The Talmud says act first, theologize later."

Giving him the confidence that he will pull through his new operation is the only way I can help Hirshel now, though I know that, starkly facing death, he is desperate for comfort.

A nurse politely but firmly asks Marcia and me to leave the room. "We have to prepare the rabbi for surgery now. You may see him again when he's ready to go to the operating room," she says to us.

When Hirshel and I went to rabbinical school in the mid-1950s, we studied the Bible in the original Hebrew, the Talmud in Aramaic, and other sacred texts of the

55

Jewish people. We also took sermonics, pastoral psychology, education, Jewish history, philosophy, and theology. We students often discussed, both inside and outside of class, the age-old theological problem of theodicy: Why is there evil and suffering in the world? Is God responsible? Can you believe in a God who allows so much evil and suffering?

The late Dr. Samuel Atlas, an intimidating man from eastern Europe, was our philosophy professor in rabbinical school. He would sit at his desk and glare at us as he lectured in his thick accent. He linked traditional Jewish religious thought with secular philosophers like Immanuel Kant, just as eight hundred years ago Moses Maimonides blended Jewish beliefs with Aristotle's philosophy. Samuel Atlas admired both Maimonides and Kant, philosophical rationalists, and considered them his spiritual mentors.

Hirshel and I got good grades in Professor Atlas's classes, but it was difficult. Dr. Atlas forced his students to be precise when talking about theology—not easy to do. In his quest for precision, the term "fuzzy" was one of Atlas's most damning terms, a description we tried to avoid at all costs.

More than a quarter of a century has passed since I sat in Dr. Atlas's classroom. There have been many changes at our rabbinical school. The Hebrew Union College has moved from its dark and dreary quarters on Manhattan's West Side to a bright, modern building in Greenwich Village. About half the rabbinical students there are now women. But I still quake when I think of Dr. Atlas, and I can still hear him making rigorous academic demands on me.

Professor Atlas relentlessly forced us to lay out the problem of theodicy clearly, unsentimentally, and without wishful thinking. He taught us to ask the right questions and not be afraid of the answers, even if they aren't what we want to hear. He forced us to go beyond easy and conventional conclusions.

While Marcia and I pace nervously in the hospital corridor, we still seek those same satisfying and consoling answers to the questions about evil and suffering that have tormented people since the beginning of time.

If there is only one God, and that God is good and all-powerful, as Jews believe, then why does the world He created have evil and suffering in it? If God is good, He would not want us to suffer. If He is all-powerful, He could prevent it. C. S. Lewis, a popular Christian writer, states the dilemma in its simplest form: "If God were good, He would wish to make His creatures perfectly happy, and if God were almighty He would be able to do what He wished. But the creatures are not happy. Therefore God lacks either goodness, or power, or both."

The Jewish tradition tries to strike a balance between complaining about suffering and meeting its challenge. Jewish law forbids us to cause pain or suffering to others, even animals, and the tradition teaches us to have compassion for those who suffer and to do all we can to alleviate their pain. When the Messiah comes, pain and suffering will be abolished. The early part of the Bible doesn't deal with the philosophical problem of evil. It assumes all God's creation is good, and any flaws in it are our fault. Later the Book of Isaiah and some psalms raise questions about evil, but the Book of Job is the only systematic attempt in the Bible to confront it.

"Job's friends told him he was suffering because of something he must have done," I say to Marcia. "Maybe pain *is* God's way of punishing us for our bad behavior."

"I don't think so. Hirshel may not be as righteous as Job was, but he couldn't have done anything to deserve

57

leukemia, Jim. That just makes us feel guilty and makes us blame ourselves. It certainly doesn't help us feel any better. What about the argument that God uses evil and suffering to teach us and make us stronger? You know that suffering builds character and Hirshel's illness is really a blessing in disguise because it will help him grow and become more compassionate. Suffering and pain enrich our lives even though we may not be able to understand this at the time."

Another version of that argument is that somehow evil will be transformed into good. The sufferings of individuals and of the Jewish people throughout its long history will be overcome and replaced with goodness, justice, and mercy. Even in the face of the murderous Crusades of the Middle Ages, the bloody Spanish Inquisition in the fifteenth and sixteenth centuries, the pogroms of Eastern Europe in the nineteenth and twentieth centuries, and the Nazi Holocaust in my lifetime, some people believe, as thirteen-year-old Anne Frank so poignantly wrote in her diary discovered after World War II, that "people are still good at heart," and that the world, despite its flaws and injustices, is basically "good at heart."

But, I wonder, what kind of God hands out such cruel punishments to good people like Hirshel Jaffe or innocents like Anne Frank and millions of other Holocaust victims? If God uses suffering for teaching, then He must be cruel, for He could certainly devise easier ways for us to learn such lessons. Besides, the "lessons" aren't handed out fairly: many good people are punished while many bad people are not and are even rewarded for their behavior. How we act often seems to make no difference. If God merely hands out suffering indiscriminately, then all we can do is scramble to escape the savagery of an angry, unforgiving, and perhaps malevolent God. Is an all-powerful God who isn't good or compassionate worthy of our worship and prayers?

Trying to justify the unequal distribution of reward and punishment, some say everything will balance out in the next life. We'll be rewarded when we die. Although Judaism emphasizes the importance of *this* life instead of an afterlife, some rabbis have taught we will be compensated for our earthly suffering in the World to Come.

"Then there's St. Augustine's solution that evil is a negation," Marcia points out. "Evil doesn't really exist —it is an illusion. Since God's creation is good, and evil is only an absence of good, God is not responsible for evil."

"Maimonides said something like that too."

"But that's just sophistry, and only explains away evil," Marcia complains. "It doesn't deal with the reality of suffering in our lives. Neither does the argument that we, not God, cause evil because of our freedom of choice. That claims it's better to have our freedom than to have a perfect world. I bet you could find a lot of people who would disagree with that! Then there are those who say we wouldn't appreciate good without the bad as a contrast. Life would be boring and meaningless . . . so what are we supposed to do, Jim, not ask questions and just have blind faith?"

"The voice in the whirlwind tells Job we can't understand God's workings and scolds him for questioning God. There is no rational solution to the problem of evil; we just have to have faith. Good and evil are human ways of thinking about things, human intellectual classifications. We see only parts of things. If we could only see things as God does, as a whole, we would realize that the whole is good, that God has reasons for giving us evil and suffering."

"Jim, these answers don't comfort us because they

don't tell us why we suffer. And they don't resolve the question of God's character—we still have to wonder if this God who makes us suffer is good. If God is so all-powerful, can't He think of other, less painful ways to make human life interesting or teach us lessons? All these 'answers' only make us ask ourselves if we can believe in a God who operates like this.

"Sometimes I think the answer that makes the most sense is the Limited God theory that Rabbi Harold Kushner wrote about. Maybe God is good but not all-powerful. Maybe He just can't do anything to stop evil and suffering just as He can't control hurricanes or earthquakes. God can't prevent things like Hirshel's leukemia because He can't intervene and suspend the laws of nature, even if He'd like to. Since God can't prevent evil, He's not responsible for it."

"But, Marcia, is this the God of the Bible? It makes you nervous—could a finite God control His own universe? Isn't God supposed to be all-powerful? Why bother at all to worship Him?"

"I know, Jim, there are problems, but there are advantages to this position too. Kushner says we become God's co-workers. We are limited, He is limited, but together as partners we can make a difference and try to overcome evil and suffering. Since God is as troubled by evil as we are, He agonizes with us and we can draw on Him for strength."

I have to agree with Marcia that this might be a more comforting God than the traditional omnipotent but possibly cruel deity. We can't blame God for evil because He is not responsible for it. So we can believe God is good and compassionate. I wonder today, waiting in this hospital corridor for Hirshel to undergo risky surgery, whether this answer to the problem of evil would bring my friend any solace.

Modern philosophers cast the problem of evil in contemporary terms. Martin Buber, the famous professor of philosophy who left his teaching position in Frankfurt, Germany, in the 1930s and moved to Jerusalem, describes evil as absence of relation and direction in our lives. The struggle against evil begins within each person; evil is redeemed by reestablishing relations with each other and with God.

From 1933 to 1945 the world witnessed the monstrous Nazi Holocaust, the deliberate, systematic, and official government murder of eleven million civilians, including six million Jews. The sheer number of victims, the carefully developed plans to expedite the killings, the length of the terror, the cold indifference of much of the "civilized" world to the Nazi plan of mass destruction, and the innocence of the victims caused many to question God. Some feel we can no longer believe in a God who allowed the Holocaust to happen.

Elie Wiesel, who survived the Auschwitz death camp, disagrees. Despair forced him to form a new relationship with God. While in the concentration camp, Weisel decided that the promise of the original Covenant is broken and now we must forge a new one. But, he urges, we cannot reject God or our religion. "We must create beauty out of nothingness. . . . We have to fight murder and absurdity and give meaning to the battle. . . ." Wiesel claims the Holocaust teaches us to lower our expectations about God. We can no longer look for Him to intervene in human history. "I no longer ask You for either happiness or paradise," Weisel tells God. "All I ask of You is to listen and let me be aware of Your listening."

The devastation of the Holocaust provides evidence for the theory our provocative Professor Atlas threw out to us in rabbinical school. Perhaps, he once lectured, there is no God, nothing to pray to, nothing to hear Hirshel's desperate plea for help. There are no ultimate answers to the problem of evil or to anything else. The entire world is simply random chance—leukemia for my friend Hirshel Jaffe, Hodgkin's disease for my brother, heart attacks for some, and long and sunlit lives for others—but all random chance.

Was Albert Einstein wrong, Dr. Atlas probed, when he declared, "God doesn't shoot dice with the universe"? Perhaps there is no God to throw the dice, and perhaps there are no dice at all. Perhaps there is only a universe of pure chance, of chaos and evil and suffering that just exists without meaning. Perhaps, as Iago proclaims in his famous "Credo" aria in Verdi's opera *Othello*, we really are simply "the sport of an unjust fate from the germ of the cradle to the worm of the grave."

"It's hard to have faith," I, the rabbi, admit to my wife.

"That's what existentialism is all about," she reminds me. "When I was in graduate school I studied Paul Tillich. He tries to come to grips with this problem by linking religious faith to our human existentialist doubt. He defines faith as 'the state of being ultimately concerned.' I wasn't sure what he meant, but I think he was saying we are being religious when we totally commit ourselves to asking meaningful questions. Faith results from—or *is*—the questions we ask, not the answers we get. There is no faith without doubt. Existential doubt and faith are two sides of the same coin, which is the process of being ultimately concerned."

"So it's the questions, not the answers, that are important?"

"Yes."

"That's very Jewish also, Marcia. Keep asking the right questions. . . ."

"Rabbi Jaffe is ready to go to the operating room now," the nurse informs us. "Perhaps you want to see him before he goes?" As Marcia and I rush back to be with our friend, a tall, good-looking man also walks into his room.

"Robert, you made it!" Hirshel says. "Jim and Marcia, this is my brother Robert."

We have never met Hirshel's other brother, Robert. We shake hands, and I tell Hirshel we're going downstairs so he and Robert can be alone together.

Hirshel looks up at me, and I can read his thoughts in his eyes. He is thinking maybe we won't ever see each other again. I don't know what to say. I put my hand on his cheek for a moment and then leave the room quickly.

We find Ronnie in the hospital waiting room. Soon Robert joins us. The two brothers have not seen each other for some time. This is obviously an intense and emotional moment for them, and Marcia and I feel like intruders.

Judi rushes into the waiting room. She greets Robert and asks what is happening. She is dismayed to find that Hirshel has already gone to the operating room, and that she didn't make it to the hospital in time to be with him.

"They took him into surgery almost immediately after I got up to his room," Robert explains. "I walked beside him as they wheeled him out. As we went through the corridors, I held his hand and told him I love him. Then they wheeled him into the operating room, but right before he disappeared through the double doors he did the most courageous thing. It was so typical of Hirshel. Even though he was heavily sedated, he raised both his fists into the air, like he was saying to me, 'I'm going to make it. I'm going to beat this!' "

6

~~~

M*y life is totally out of my control.*
    Three days since the second operation, and they're still not sure if it worked.

At least I lived through it. I know it was a close call. The surgeon told Judi when he came out of the operating room that it was a very tricky operation and he was really sweating it. My bowel had become gangrenous, necrotic, because it wasn't being used. He had to cut out the dead part. And he was worried he might have to do further surgery if it didn't work.

Today is the first day they can try to give me something to drink. But it is very complicated. The nurses have to unclamp my stomach every two or three hours to see if I can take a few ounces of liquid. It's like my whole life depends on whether or not I can take these one or two ounces!

And the confusion you see in a hospital doesn't make you feel any better. Last night the nurse mixed up my urine chart with my roommate's, who had kidney stones. I woke up and saw her entering my urine output onto his chart. And when I went down for an X-ray after the surgery, the radiologist said, "Frankly, Rabbi, some people just don't have a lot of luck." That really cheered me up! Then I overheard the physicians toying with the idea of making a cut in my neck to put my IV in because they were running out of places to put it in my arms. I just couldn't stand the thought of that!

But the worst thing happened today. When my parents arrived—thank God they finally got here—and asked the hematologist if the surgery had worked, I heard him say sarcastically, "Dr. and Mrs. Jaffe, we don't know. Maybe he'll need three or four or five more operations." I couldn't believe he had said that. I said to my parents, "Did you hear that?" I don't think physicians realize how patients hang on their every word and how devastating an offhand comment like that can be.

Of course, I've become a little cynical about doctors since I've been here. I've been in the hospital so long and I see what's going on. Yesterday a physician came in to see my roommate. (God, I've had so many roommates come and go, and I'm still here. That makes me feel worse.) My roommate was sleeping, or else he was just out of it, because the doctor was talking to him, asking him how he felt, but he didn't answer back.

So I hear the doctor sort of carrying on a conversation with himself, answering his own questions, like he's really talking to my roommate. I heard the whole thing, and I couldn't believe it. I couldn't resist saying something to the physician. I wanted to let him know I had caught him at it. So right before he left the room, I said to him, "Well, that was the easiest seventy-five dollars you ever made for a hospital visit, wasn't it?" I think he was shocked. I'm sure he didn't realize I was even there. I guess they'll be glad to see me leave here —if I ever do. The whole hospital staff will probably have a party when Rabbi Jaffe leaves!

I'm surprised I can even joke. My spirits are pretty low.

August 30, 1982

I am going home tomorrow! I can't believe it!

Four days ago my surgeon came into my room, and I guess seeing all the mismanagement and confusion and slipups, he

66

suddenly said to a nurse, "Tear down Rabbi Jaffe's charts."
He ripped them off the end of my bed and said, "Take these
away. Take out his IVs and start giving him liquids. I know
he's going to make it."

It wasn't a strict scientific medical decision on his part. It
was more an act of faith, and his act of faith gave me faith.
I've never felt more elated, because immediately after that I
started to feel like the old Hirshel again.

The effect of my surgeon's words reminded me of something
that happened a few years ago. I went to a hospital to visit a
man in my congregation who had been in a coma for a week.
He had had a stroke, and they were ready to give him up. The
family was already asking me about his funeral. It was a
Friday evening, right before Sabbath services, and I walked
into his room, and just out of impulse I said, "Good Shabbas,
Samuel." His eyes fluttered, and he looked up, and he said,
"Good Shabbas, Rabbi." The family thought I was a miracle
worker. He had a few more precious hours of communication
with his loved ones, and then he died.

This kind of thing has happened to me more than once as
a rabbi. Of course, these people have revived only briefly. I've
never healed anyone; I don't believe in that. But it shows how
important faith is. I have imagined that I'm battling my
cancer cells. They say that's supposed to help kill them. I don't
know if there's anything to that, but I know my mental out-
look is very important, more now than ever before. A coura-
geous attitude can make all the difference, and my surgeon's
act of faith in tearing down those charts gave me courage
because then I knew that I'd make it.

Right after that I began to take liquids and then forty-eight
hours later soft food, and finally my intestines began to work.
It was like a miracle. Boy, we really take our body for granted
until something goes wrong. Jews recite an important daily
morning prayer thanking God for keeping our bodily orifices
in working order. We say, "Blessed art Thou, O Lord our God,

King of the Universe, Who has formed man in wisdom and created in him many passages and vessels . . . if but one of these be opened, or one of these be closed, it would be impossible to exist and stand before Thee. Blessed art Thou, O Lord, Who art the wondrous Healer of all flesh." Judaism never minimizes or disparages our routine bodily functions. It celebrates and sanctifies them because the tradition keeps reminding us that we owe our health to God, and that our bodies as well as our souls reflect His creation.

Yesterday Judi brought in my favorite silky blue Adidas running suit and said, "Hirshel, get out of that awful hospital gown and put this on. You're a human being again." So I put it on, and immediately I felt better, and I've been walking around the halls, like I am doing laps. I'm talking to other patients, like a chaplain. I guess I'm finally reentering the world. I'm reasserting my old identity.

I'm doing so well they said I can go home tomorrow. At last. I can hardly believe it.

August 31, 1982

I am home! It's really wonderful.

All the way home in the car I kept thinking, "I made it, I made it."

This afternoon as I was watching Judi drive me home, I thought for the first time about all she has endured while I was in the hospital. I have been too concerned about myself to think about what Judi's had to cope with. She's been under tremendous pressure. I don't know how she handled it.

She drove more than one hundred miles back and forth to the hospital to see me almost every day. Then when she got home at night, so exhausted, she was besieged by phone calls from relatives and friends and congregants wanting to know how I was. People telephone incessantly. She feels she has to talk to everyone who calls. And I telephoned her every night and unloaded all my latest aches and pains and fears on her. I must have driven her crazy.

She's had to contend with the whole family—my parents, her mother—and deal with Rachel's and Nina's anxieties. They say, "Daddy's sick, you mean I can't have what I want?" The only time she's had to relax is during the hour's drive to and from the hospital. She listened to country music and used that time to try to pull herself together for the next day when everything started over again. She told me, "Hirshel, it's as if for me there was no summer."

And she knows she has to go back to her demanding job soon. She hasn't felt well herself this summer. She has a pounding, pulsating pain in her neck, and her stomach is acting up. The stress is taking a toll on her body.

It's been hard for Judi as a nurse because she can see what goes on in hospitals. She knew that things were going wrong. She knew my life was in their hands when she left there every night, and she was worried. But she realized if she interfered it could hurt me. The staff might say, "OK, if you're so smart, Mrs. Jaffe, you do it."

And like many other wives she's totally unprepared to become a widow. While I was in the hospital, she was filling out insurance forms and car registration forms and all those things for the first time in her life. She's been overwhelmed with details and paperwork on top of everything else.

Today after I got home Judi gave me the pile of cards and letters that came to the house while I was in the hospital. There are hundreds of them. I read them today for the first time. They aren't just greeting cards. Most people wrote their own letters. I got messages from people I never knew had such depth and cared so much. I can see the effort they put into writing them. I realize now that people are capable of a lot more thoughtfulness and feeling than you might imagine.

Almost every personal card or letter from congregants re-

calls something I have done to touch them, like console them or visit them in the hospital. I realized as I read the cards how much as a rabbi I've affected people's lives. It's rare to learn that except when you're ill and people make an effort to tell you.

One particular letter really moved me. It came from a woman in Philadelphia who reminded me that years ago when I was a student rabbi there I worked with a group of retarded children, one of whom was her daughter, Laura. I taught the children to say the "Sh'ma," touch the Torah, things like that. It took a lot of patience. Before I left the congregation, the six retarded children and teenagers wrote their signatures and they were embossed on a letterhead that said, "To Rabbi Jaffe with Love." One of those names is that of little Laura, the daughter of the woman who wrote me the letter. That letterhead still sits on my desk in my study at the temple. I think I cherish that more than any other memento.

These letters give me hope and encourage me. When you're down you should turn from your depression and just remember all those things that are the best part of yourself and aim for that. Like that letterhead with the children's names: now when I look at it on my desk, it will give me strength because it reminds me of the good I'm capable of doing.

"Things are settling down into a routine," Hirshel tells me when I telephone him about a week after he gets out of the hospital. "Rachel and Nina are back in school, and Judi has started teaching again. The college couldn't give her any more time off. The nuns were very understanding and made concessions to her about summer obligations and preparation, but now reality has set in and she had to go back to work.

"Oh, Jim, I have to tell you what Judi did. It's so

funny, but it might set the cause of Jewish-Christian relations back a hundred years. It was so hot in Judi's little office at Mount St. Mary that one of the students she was counseling there nearly fainted. It was about ninety-five degrees. Judi has begged them over and over again for an electric fan to cool her office. She says everybody else has a fan. Well, she got desperate and decided to do something drastic.

"She went down to the front of the chapel and took the little statue of the Virgin Mary from the pedestal and hid it in her office. She left a note where the statue had stood, saying, 'When you give me a fan so I can breathe, you will get your statue back.'

"The whole place was in an uproar, but it worked. She got her fan in twenty minutes. They all laughed. They love Judi there. She's very popular. She's great with the nursing students, so caring. And it's such a joke around there that here's a rabbi's wife teaching in a Catholic college with all the nuns and priests. The nuns are praying for me, by the way. That's touching."

"How are you, Hirshel? Are you gaining your strength back?"

"I'm feeling a little stronger every day. But I am getting some more abdominal pain and spasms. The doctors say they're nothing to worry about. But I'm afraid to eat anything, and I'm not putting on any weight, which is bad. And I'm still taking pills so I can sleep. I'm afraid I'm relying on them too much.

"It's great being out of the hospital. But you know, Jim, I'm lonely here in the house all day, and I still feel like a prisoner. Judi and the girls are busy with their own lives. I know this sounds self-centered, but things seem to be a bit anticlimactic now. I used to complain in the hospital that the staff never left me alone. But I guess I miss all the attention. It's hard not having Judi here to

71

cater to me and cheer me up. When I asked, 'Who'll get my meals for me?' she said with her dry humor, 'You will, Hirshel.' I'll have to learn not to be so dependent on her now.

"Maybe it will be better when I get more energy and can leave the house. When you are used to being active all day, it's hard to lie around and do nothing. It's one thing being in the hospital. You know you can't do anything there, and somehow you just accept it. But when you're home you feel you ought to be doing something useful. I feel guilty because I'm not doing much. And I feel like the world is passing me by.

"Thank God for my visitors. It's like therapy to talk to them. They are giving me such support. Father Fenlon comes over to see me. He's a very special priest. He went to Israel recently and wrote a prayer for me on a little piece of paper and put it in the Western Wall in Jerusalem. He spoke about our friendship at a Shabbas service at my synagogue. Rabbi Steve Arnold from Poughkeepsie comes over all the time. He's like my rabbi in a way. He's so kind and wise. And I get a lot of telephone calls.

"My running buddies stop by every morning to see me when they jog up our hill. We all used to run together every morning before we went to work. I know they mean well, but it's agonizing for me to see them running when I can't. One morning they ran up our hill and yelled out, 'Come on, Hirshel,' and I actually stumbled out onto the porch with my sneakers on, like we were going to run together like in the old days."

"What about the High Holidays, Hirshel? Will you be able to officiate?"

"I was hoping I would be able to do the services. But I've learned by now that you can't always dictate to your body. I won't have the energy. My congregants don't want me to push myself, so they invited Rabbi Herbert Drooz from Delaware to help with the services. He's retired now. I told my president I'll participate as much as I can. He said I should take it easy as long as I need to.

"I'm lucky, my congregants have been so understanding. They told me not to worry about anything. But how long are they going to tolerate my lying around like this, not being able to work? Conducting High Holiday services is one of our main jobs. Something is really wrong when the rabbi misses them. We always complain about how much work the Holidays are and how we'll never make it through them, but they are such an important part of our lives."

"Hirshel, I always say the High Holidays are like a bell that rings, and, like race horses, we rabbis are off and running. . . ."

The approach of the High Holidays in early autumn is an anxious time for rabbis. They are the holiest days in the Jewish calendar, and they come all at once after the summer lull. It is a congregational rabbi's busiest season, with the largest crowds of the year. First comes Rosh Hashana, the New Year, and then ten days later the Day of Atonement. During those ten days there is a special Sabbath, and on the Sunday between Rosh Hashana and Yom Kippur many congregations hold memorial services at their cemeteries. Sukkot, the harvest Festival of Tabernacles, comes five days after Yom Kippur, and we conclude the entire Holiday season a week later with the celebration of Simchat Torah, when we joyously carry the Torah scrolls around the synagogue and begin the weekly Torah reading cycle all over again.

All these holidays involve special and often very long worship services, and we must prepare many sermons on a wide range of subjects. The High Holiday season heavily taxes a rabbi's physical and psychic energy. Yom Kippur is especially exhausting, since most Jews do not eat or drink anything on this holy day of repentance. The High Holidays also coincide with the beginning of religious school and all the synagogue's regular activities the rabbi supervises. The pressure of the High Holiday season is difficult for every congregational rabbi. It has been called a rabbi's endurance test, a kind of marathon race.

For Hirshel, who has just stared death in the face, the High Holidays of 1982 will be especially gripping because of their powerful spiritual message. The High Holidays are a time for searching our souls and talking about our personal relationship to God. We deal with our dependence on God, such basic concepts as sin and repentance, and we confront our own mortality. The Day of Atonement is not connected to a specific historical event—it has to do with the shortcomings and vulnerabilities of being human. It's like looking into our personal mirror free of our ordinary posturing, posing, defenses, perhaps the only time during the year when we are completely honest with ourselves. We might run from our inner selves all year, but during the High Holidays the running and hiding are supposed to stop.

This year I will lead High Holiday services in the Pennsylvania leisure community where we have our vacation home. The synagogue building is a wooden one-room structure that seems to nestle subtly in the surrounding mountains and trees. Sometimes during the services through the large front windows you can see deer pick their way delicately through the forest. You really think about God and the miracle of creation in that beautiful mountain setting. I like to officiate at High Holiday services; because of my work at the American

Jewish Committee I don't perform the ceremonial duties of a congregational rabbi often, except for an occasional wedding or, sadly, funeral.

Every year at this time I go through a sort of spiritual reappraisal of myself. It's refreshing to take time out from a busy schedule, to give myself over to self-reflection. When Marcia and Eve and Jennifer complain they can't pursue their normal activities during the Holidays, I always tell them, "You can work or play on other days of the year. Use these few days to take stock of your lives."

This year the Holidays will take on a special dimension for me because of my friend Hirshel's illness. Of course, the uncertainty of Hirshel's fate is true for all of us. Something like Hirshel's leukemia could hit any of us tomorrow. How can we know what lies ahead? One of my friends compares the unpredictability of life to a lottery. Is existence pure chance, or is there a plan or meaning? It is this uncertainty of existence, the vulnerability of all human beings, that makes the High Holy Days so compelling, even riveting.

According to Jewish tradition, on Rosh Hashana God decides who will live and who will die in the new year by entering our names into the Book of Life. On Yom Kippur the Book of Life is closed for twelve months. During the High Holiday services Jews read a prayer called the "Unetaneh Tokef," recited centuries ago by a martyred rabbi shortly before he was put to death during the Crusades. This prayer poetically expresses our realization of the precariousness of life and our desire to believe that our destinies are controlled by God:

> As the shepherd seeks out his flock,
> and makes the sheep pass under his staff,

so do You muster and number and consider every soul,
setting the bounds of every creature's life,
and decreeing its destiny.

On Rosh Hashana it is written,
on Yom Kippur it is sealed:
How many shall pass on, how many shall come to be;
who shall live and who shall die;
who shall see ripe age and who shall not;
who shall perish by fire and who by water;
who by sword and who by beast;
who by hunger and who by thirst;
who by earthquake and who by plague;
who by strangling and who by stoning;
who shall be secure and who shall be driven;
who shall be tranquil and who shall be troubled;
who shall be poor and who shall be rich;
who shall be humbled and who exalted.

I think of my older brother, Bert, dead for eight years,
and now I think of Hirshel, and the prayer hits me personally as never before. For years I have recited these
words, but they never really entered my heart as they
will this year.

Probably every rabbi has heard the question, "Why
should I continue to recite prayers if the words don't
really mean much to me? Why say them over and over
if they don't touch me personally?" The Jewish tradition
has answered this important question in an intriguing
way.

One of the best-known prayers in our liturgy comes
from the Book of Deuteronomy: "And you shall love the
Lord, your God. . . . Set these words, which I command
you this day, upon your heart." Why, the Biblical commentators ask, does the prayer say to set God's words
"upon your heart," and not "in your heart"? The answer
is that prayers often lie fallow upon a person's heart

waiting only for the heart to open and become receptive to their meaning. When a person's heart is finally ready to receive the prayers, the words, already waiting symbolically in place "upon the heart," suddenly rush into the person's consciousness like a flood of water, sometimes with overwhelming power. That is exactly what the "Unetaneh Tokef" has done to me this year.

Rosh Hashana

It was strange and painful seeing somebody else up in my pulpit last night and today, but I also felt so much more, so many positive emotions that I hadn't expected.

Judi bundled me up and helped me into the car, and she purposely arrived late at the Rosh Hashana services last night to shield me from the large crowd. I appeared in the congregation just at the point when the cantor was concluding the blessing with the words "Shehecheyanu," a prayer of thanks to God for keeping us alive and letting us reach this day. There was a real stir in the sanctuary; I guess my congregants realized the significance of this prayer for me. I certainly did.

How many times in my life have I recited the words of the "Shehecheyanu" prayer—"Blessed is the Lord our God, Ruler of the universe, for keeping us alive, for sustaining us, and for letting us reach this day"—without thinking too much about them. But last night as we said those words I realized we ought to be more conscious of the miracle of life.

I also thought about the fact that the "Shehecheyanu" prayer is written in the plural. It's "Blessed art Thou, O God, who has kept us alive and sustained us and enabled us to reach this day." It doesn't say, "Kept me alive." I don't think the plural form is an accident. The authors wanted us to realize that survival is communal. We can't make it alone in this life. Somebody did a survey not long ago and found that people who live alone have shorter lives. We need the emotional support system of family, friends, and community. I never could have come through this without everybody's help.

Later on in the service when they opened the ark that holds the Torah scroll and the cantor sang the "Avinu Malkenu," I really started trembling. What a powerful prayer, and how it spoke to me tonight! "Our Father, our King, hear our voice; Our Father, our King, we have sinned against You; Our Father, our King, have compassion on us and on our children; Our Father, our King, make an end to sickness, war, and famine; Our Father, our King, make an end to all oppression; Our Father, our King, inscribe us for blessing in the Book of Life. . . ." Does God really inscribe us in a book of life? Is our fate really sealed? Is everything decided for us? Have I made it into the Book of Life for another year?

I know scholars have debated the meaning of this prayer for centuries. I feel uncomfortable telling people our destinies are preordained because Judaism also teaches that God created us with a free will. I believe God is the ultimate master of our lives, but He works in partnership with us, and we must actively influence our own fate as much as possible. So the outcome of my leukemia is not predestined, and I'll go on fighting as long as I can.

Since I wasn't busy officiating today, I could really concentrate on the words of the prayer book. I kept thinking how relevant the prayers are to me. How the deep mystery of the ever-renewing cycle of life, the birthday of the world which Rosh Hashana celebrates—mythologically anyway—is so meaningful to me now that my life may be shortened.

As the beautiful liturgy says, "Your blessing glows in every spark of time. Again and again the morning stars unite to hymn Your love. Again the sun comes forth to sing Your light. Again the angels sing their sacred chant to You. Again souls intone their need for You. Again the grasses sing their thirst for You. Again the birds chirp their joy before You." Again and again and again, the poetry repeats. Again . . . forever. Yes, I kept thinking, even if I do die, the world and life will go on, year after year. There is a continuity of nature and a continuity of creation even in death, and that is strangely comforting.

And of course the moment of the "Unetanah Tokef" prayer was staggering to me. I said to myself, "Who shall live? I shall live!" I shall live to see my daughters grow older. It isn't fair —my girls are only nine and eleven. I shall live to see Nina win more ribbons for her horseback riding and Rachel become a Bat Mitzvah in a year and a half!

The "Unetanah Tokef" says God decides not only who shall live and who shall die, but also what kind of year we'll have. "Who shall be secure and who shall be driven? Who shall be tranquil and who shall be troubled?" I thought carefully about those words "tranquil" and "troubled" when we all recited the prayer together. In Hebrew they are spelled identically except for one letter. This shows what a thin line in life there is between trouble and tranquillity.

Even if I do live, my life won't be as peaceful or secure as it was before. I'll always be worried about my leukemia coming back. Every time I get a cold or a little flu, I'll wonder if an infection will bring me down. I'll be worried about Judi and the girls trying to make it financially if I can't work or if I die. I have to think about these huge medical bills piling up. I worry about Judi trying to raise two daughters alone. . . . Yes, I'll be driven and troubled.

But the most moving moment came at the end of the evening service last night when Rabbi Drooz called on me to help him give the congregation the closing blessing. I slowly walked through the sanctuary, climbed the stairs to the pulpit carefully, and stood beside Herb. There was total silence. Hundreds of people stared at me.

We both lifted our hands to pronounce the blessing, and my mind flashed back to that day in the hospital a couple of weeks *ago when I was so sick and Marty Freedman came to visit me. I had said to him, "Give me your blessing," and he lifted up his hands and blessed me. And now I was lifting up my hands to bless my congregation.*

7

∿∿∿

September 28, 1982

F*our days ago there was a horrible fire at the house of a family in my congregation. Both parents died. The twelve-year-old boy ran back into the house and crawled on his hands and knees and saved his little sister. His Bar Mitzvah is coming up in a few months. That will be devastating now that his parents are dead.*

The temple was packed with hundreds of stunned mourners, and I officiated at their funeral only a few hours before the start of Yom Kippur. Everyone was asking why these people died so senselessly. I felt frail and weak, but somehow I got through it. It must have been obvious to everyone what an ordeal it was for me. Afterward one of my congregants came to help me down the stairs from the pulpit. He reached out and embraced me and said, "Rabbi, you have comforted these people so well. But who shall comfort the comforter?"

It was a beautiful expression of concern for me. And it's a good question.

October 2, 1982

It feels so great to be running again. Last week when I was able to run my first mile I actually cried. I came back home, took off my sweats, and looked in the mirror. I said in front of the mirror, in tears, "I did it, I did it, I did it."

Of course, I may never run as far or as fast as I did before. People are always asking me if I'm running again. I tell them I'm running more with my heart than with my feet. I know my limitations.

I was foolish to think because I ran I'd live forever. No more pacts with God while I'm running on South Beach. I see now how presumptuous I was. I'm more realistic now. I'm running more for my head than for exercise now.

October 4, 1982

Flew out to Chicago yesterday to see the leading expert in hairy-cell leukemia. When I had my spleenectomy, Judi kept asking the physicians, "Who knows the most about Hirshel's disease?" She kept after them until they gave her the name of this man. I'm lucky she was so persistent. She wants to make sure I have the best care possible.

I was surprised to see how young this specialist is. Only in his early forties and already head of his department. He's obviously brilliant. He's ebullient too, good at lifting a patient's spirits.

When he looked at my records and saw I'm a rabbi, he said, "My son is becoming a Bar Mitzvah soon." He asked me a lot of questions about my running. He told me he wants to lose some weight and asked me how to start jogging.

He is wonderfully supportive. He was confident after the painful bone marrow examination that I'll have a long remission. I returned home elated, but somehow Judi seems to be shielding herself. She's not as optimistic as I am.

Last week I was resting at home when suddenly I heard a van pull into our driveway. I looked out the window and saw Myron and some other friends from the congregation unload something from the van. I ran outside. They were starting to build a sukkah* right in our backyard to help us celebrate Sukkot. It was a complete surprise. I couldn't believe it.*

Myron works in the carpet business, and he used those big, empty carpet tubes as the framework for the little hut. Then they put leaves and cornstalks on the tubes to make the shelter. It was very clever.

Then the next night my orthodox rabbi friend brought over a lulav* and* etrog* for me to hold and wave in praise of God's goodness for keeping me alive. It was a wonderful symbol of friendship to me.*

October 18, 1982

I'm slowly but surely getting back to work. It's hard. I realize now I may never have the energy I did before. My stomach is giving me trouble. I have to watch what I eat. And I have to stop taking all these damned pills the doctor prescribed. But I push myself and work as much as I can. My

---

sukkah: The temporary booth erected during the week-long fall harvest festival of Sukkot to commemorate the ancient Israelites' wanderings in the wilderness following the Exodus from Egypt.

lulav: A cluster of palm, myrtle, and willow branches shaken during Sukkot, symbolizing the autumn harvest.

etrog: A yellow citrus fruit whose aroma symbolizes the sweetness of the autumn harvest during Sukkot.

physicians told me it's good therapy to get back to work as soon as possible.

I guess I'm trying to prove to myself that I can function. I think if I'm working well, I must feel well. And working does help me feel better, as the doctors said it would. It takes me out of myself. It lifts my spirits, and I think I am almost conquering the disease.

It's interesting—the Hebrew word for "sick" comes from the word chalah, *which means emptiness. But a healthy person is a* bah-ree, *from the word* bah-rah, *which means "to create." A healthy person is one that can create or work; the unhealthy person's life is empty because he's not productive.*

It's amazing how much insight the Bible has about human nature. The writers obviously realized how valuable work is for a person's self-esteem. The work ethic has always been important in Judaism. Work was given as a covenant by God, just as the Torah was. Even God worked when He created the world! Work is so important in Judaism that we shouldn't look down on any type of labor. You should work not only to support yourself but to keep out of trouble. I remember one Talmudic scholar warned us that idleness causes bad things.

Working really does help you keep your mind off your illness. A couple of years ago I preached a sermon on Norman Cousins' book about his illness. He writes about how he felt so much better when he brought his work to the hospital, even though at first the hospital staff didn't like it. He believes creativity helps cure illness. Cousins tells this incredible story about a time he visited Pablo Casals when the great musician was in his late eighties. Casals' body was all stooped, and his hands curled up, and he was in unbearable pain. But when he sat down at his cello or at the piano, his spine and fingers mysteriously straightened and he was able to play magnificently and overcome his pain. When he was immersed in his work, his great art, the pain disappeared.

Of course I have to pace myself. So I choose my priorities more carefully now. My congregation doesn't let me overdo it. Somebody has taken over my confirmation class, and there is even talk about getting me an assistant rabbi. I know this leukemia has shaken my people. I can tell some of them are ambivalent about my illness. It's been hard for them because now they realize I have serious problems to cope with like everybody else. They can see that the leader of the flock can't always lead and now sometimes needs a shepherd of his own to guide him.

Sometimes my congregants make me feel I'm failing them because they expect me to be a cheerleader for everybody like I always was. Before I came back to work, one man said, "Oh, Rabbi, it's not the same when you're not here to conduct services. We feel rudderless." Of course he was only trying to compliment me, but that made me feel bad because I wasn't up to it.

I feel I have to muster up my energy and put on an act— hide my illness and make my voice sound lively—so I can give them hope. My congregants would be dismayed if they knew they were making it difficult for me because they want to help me so much, but it's becoming a problem that I can't escape. I feel I have to live up to their expectations of me. I don't express my true feelings because I don't want them to know how scared and worried I really am.

Some of my congregants have been almost apologetic because of my illness. They hate to burden me with their problems, and they're anxious about me and oversolicitous. It's funny—they tell me conflicting things. One person will say, "Gee, you look great," and on the same day another person will tell me, "You look tired, Rabbi—go home and get some rest."

It's tough to answer people honestly when they send me such mixed messages. Sometimes I'll say something like, "Don't worry, I know. Believe me, I'm being careful with my health."

But other times I either ignore the comment or answer vaguely because I've just heard the opposite thing five minutes before. Yet when I do that, I feel bad because I know they are trying to look out for me and they are genuinely concerned. This confusion only compounds my feelings of inadequacy. I'm haunted as a rabbi by having to be all things to all people.

It's painful now to carry out some of my rabbinic duties because I am so close to the situations I used to deal with in a more detached way. A few days ago I went to the hospital to see a congregant who has cancer. He's only forty-five years old. Well, I saw him and I kept my composure, but while I was driving home I thought, "We have the same disease, we're nearly the same age, just a few short weeks ago I was lying in the hospital!" It was like a mirror, a reverse image of what I've just gone through—lying there all day, all alone, waiting for someone to telephone me or come to see me, and terrified by all the cold, impersonal hospital procedures. It was very difficult for me to make that visit, but I knew I had to do it. I have to return to real life.

And on Yom Kippur, even though Herb Drooz was there to take over for me, I felt I had to read the list of the congregation's deceased at the memorial service. Drooz is a lovely man, but he didn't know the people who had died. I said to myself, "Hirshel, get up there and read the names." I wanted to do it because I had been part of their lives, I had consoled their families, and they are all doing so much for me now. So I got up and read the names.

I knew I had done the right thing. But reading the names of people who have died since last year's High Holidays was a very emotional experience for me because I know next year I might be on that Yahrzeit list. Another rabbi might be reading my name next year and the years after that, and I won't be here. Every week at the end of the Sabbath service when I read the names of the dead I confront the fact that my name could soon be on that list . . . nothing left of me except

*my name and fading images in my family's and friends'
memories.*

November 20, 1982

*It took me until November to convince my doctors some-
thing was really wrong with my stomach. I could hardly eat
anything by then. Right after a Bar Mitzvah I had a terrible
attack. My parents happened to be visiting us, and they drove
me to the hospital. My digestive system was partially blocked
up again, and I had to be fed intravenously for ten days. I
came home from the hospital last week.*

*I was just beginning to get some of my energy back and
work full-time, and then, boom, there I was vulnerable again
and back in the hospital. I felt like I had to climb the mountain all over again. I felt the doctors had let me down once
more. And to make matters worse, my blood counts are slipping again.*

*By now I should have realized the doctors don't know every-
thing. You can't wait for them to act; you have to take charge.
I'm an assertive person, and still I have trouble getting the
right medical attention, so you really have to wonder what
kind of care is received by people who are in awe of their
doctors and trying to be "nice." But some things are just out
of your hands. When I try to assert myself, some doctors tell
me I'm doing the right thing. They say you shouldn't jeopar-
dize your life just because you want to be polite. But if you
overdo it, the physicians think you don't trust them. You can
break the doctor-patient relationship.*

*At times I think I'm too actively trying to stage-manage my
recovery. I'm trying to get my doctors together and coordinate
them, but it's very frustrating. I realize now that I can't do it
all myself. You can't plan for everything in life. A friend of
mine told me you have to accept your vulnerability. Maybe you*

87

have to allow for your fragility and not spend every ounce of energy fighting as you would to finish a marathon race.

It was strange to see how my congregants reacted to my rehospitalization. Some said, "See, Rabbi, you overdid it, you worked too hard, it must have been something you did." And some of them felt guilty when they heard about it. They thought they had overworked me.

❦

Hirshel phones to tell us Judi is going to be in the annual Mount St. Mary variety show put on by the students and faculty. She's going to be Dolly Parton. He says Judi has been practicing Parton's hit song "My D-i-v-o-r-c-e" for weeks and has perfected her country accent. We can't miss this performance, so we drive up to Newburgh.

Judi struts out onto the stage in a blond wig, low-cut, tight dress, and spangled boots. She is very well-endowed and needs only the blond wig to transform her into the buxom country music star. The second Judi gets out onstage, even before she begins her song, pandemonium breaks out in the theater. We couldn't stop laughing. The hysterical laughter drowned out Judi's song. Later she said she was upset because she had rehearsed so much and nobody could hear her sing.

It's good to see Hirshel laughing again.

A few weeks later we drive up to Newburgh again to help Hirshel celebrate the twentieth anniversary of his ordination as a rabbi. During the service I thought, "Well, we've made it this far with Hirshel." It hasn't been easy for any of us.

It's been painful living through this ordeal with him.

And now that Hirshel's blood counts are going down again, he needs our help and encouragement more than ever. I hope we can keep it up. It's hard to be a friend at a difficult time like this. Sometimes you just want to run the other way. Yet I know I can't ignore Hirshel's problems; I have to keep on being a friend because Hirshel needs me so much now.

Hirshel used to run his marathon races alone; now we have to summon our own energy to keep running with him.

Our family just got back from a weekend in Manhattan, one of those hotel package deals at the Grand Hyatt. We had a great time. Went to the theater to see Brighton Beach Memoirs. *Fabulous. It brought back a lot of memories for me because I was born in Brighton Beach. We ate at Tavern on the Green and walked around the city to show Rachel and Nina the sights and the beautiful holiday decorations.*

Judi encouraged me to walk a lot. She bought me a rabbit fur hat because it was so cold. She kept saying, "Don't be lazy, Hirshel, now you have this warm hat, let's walk." She knows I am still leery about exerting myself. I was hesitant about making the trip at all. I didn't want to travel too far. But Judi cajoled me into it. She said, "You have to start living again, Hirshel." She packed me in the car and forced me to go places as soon as I got out of the hospital. Judi's been trying to get me to be more daring.

I'm glad now, because she's right. And we had a wonderful family time together. It was the first time the girls have seen me relaxed and "normal" since all this started last July. I forgot about my illness for a little while.

My prisoners at Greenhaven seem so concerned about me. Like that big get-well card with all their signatures they sent me when I was in the hospital last summer. Here are these guys—very hardened criminals, some of them. Murderers, rapists, the whole bit, not the world's nicest people. But they must have a little soft spot because when I visit them they always ask me how I feel, and I know they really mean it.

I guess my work with these prisoners has had some effect, though I'm so often filled with doubt. It makes me realize why I've kept this prison chaplaincy. Sometimes I've asked myself, "Is this worthwhile? What am I doing here?" Some congregants want me to give it up now that I'm ill. They're worried about the extra strain it puts on me.

It's very tough duty, emotionally draining. Not too many chaplains want to serve here. It's not a pleasant place, and almost impossible to avoid conflict. The inmates take out all their frustrations on me because I'm the chaplain, and they get angry when I can't perform miracles for them. It can be dangerous here too. One disturbed guy did scare me—the other prisoners had to calm him down. An inmate brutally murdered a woman guard right next door to the Jewish chapel.

There's so much to do here, and the prison bureaucracy doesn't make things easy. Greenhaven has the largest concentration of Jewish prisoners—about forty—in the United States. The name of the group is Congregation Hatikvah, which means "hope." On the wall of the small chapel there is a painting of hands breaking chains. An inscription on the picture, a quotation from the prayer book, reads, "He frees those who are bound."

The prisoners besiege me with requests. I perform all the Jewish rites, conduct services, counsel the inmates, make phone calls for them, write letters asking for clemency, organize volunteer groups to visit the prison, and get them kosher food. But I can see now I've touched them, after all. Has it taken my illness for me to know that? Did I have to get sick for the inmates to discover they can care about someone? Maybe those who say there is meaning in suffering because you learn from it and because it brings out the best in you and in others are right. I'd feel better knowing there is some good reason for this leukemia.

January 21, 1983

We flew up to Martha's Vineyard yesterday!

Judi took the initiative, as usual. Leave it to her to do something crazy like that. Yesterday was a beautiful day, in the fifties with bright sunshine. Judi drove to Marine Air Terminal next to LaGuardia, and she said, "Hirshel, we're going to Martha's Vineyard. I want you to know that you can make it up there." It seemed so crazy, but it meant so much to me to get back there. So we flew up. I got really emotional when we landed. Judi thought I was overdoing it, but she understood. All the time I kept thinking, "I've made it back to the Vineyard."

Everything was just as I remembered it. There were the dunes and the bike paths, the boats and our house at South Beach. The house is closed up for the winter, so we spent the night at the Charlotte Inn in Edgartown. The fire was marvelous.

It was a beautiful twenty-four hours. A time for love.

February 15, 1983

I think some of my congregants are beginning to run out of patience. They want me to be able to work as hard as I did

91

before I got sick. They see I'm in remission, and they don't realize I'm still weak. Most of them are still very understanding, but a lot of feelings have built up. About a week ago I got the word from the board. They said, "Listen, Hirshel, you really have to be more visible now." I guess the sympathy vote is over.

I don't want to worry my congregation so I don't tell them every little detail about my blood tests, all the ups and downs, but they're constantly on the lookout for signs of the illness. They comment on how pale I am. I know they are always watching me, and that's a funny feeling.

They assess my health by how high I can lift the Torah scroll up over my head in the service when we say, "This is the Torah that God gave to Moses and the people of Israel." It's the most exciting moment of the service for many of my people. But now sometimes I can almost hear them holding their breath and gasping and thinking, "Will he make it this time?"

It's lucky for me the president of the congregation is in my corner. He told me some people were saying, "What if the rabbi goes down the tube? Maybe we should organize a search committee to start looking for a new rabbi." He said to them, "Look, the rabbi is sick, he gets better, he might get sick again, but this is our rabbi." One of my friends suggested I should announce to them I'm not planning to die imminently.

I may not be doing the quantity of work I could before I got sick, but I think the quality of my work is much better. I don't waste time on silly things like making sure I smile at all the right people. Now I use that time to counsel people or visit a home for the elderly. I'm trying to make my rabbinate more personal. I want to pay more attention to my congregants' problems and give them more spiritual guidance.

People come in for counseling because they're upset or depressed, or they've had a career or business reversal, or they have problems with children or with their marriages, and now I'm able to give advice with more force and insight. Now I say things right out. A few weeks ago one of the nicest women in my congregation complained to me about her husband's abuse. Before my illness I would have just sympathized with her, but now I said, "You shouldn't take this. Don't allow yourself to be degraded and exploited. Start learning to stand up for yourself, and don't lose your dignity." I told her you have only one life, and you have to make the best of it.

Sometimes I can't help relating my congregants' problems to my own. That can be awkward. Recently a congregant told me he was hiding his liver disease because he was afraid he'd lose his job if people found out he was sick, but he was destroying himself in the process by keeping so much bottled up. I admitted, "I know what you mean, sometimes I'm afraid I'll lose my job because I'm sick." I have to be more careful. I can't cross over the line while I'm counseling people and become absorbed in my own self-pity. That only confuses people. I can't let my illness get in the way, and I can't get so preoccupied with myself that I can no longer help others.

My congregants can see that I am learning to live with my illness. Maybe that helps them cope better with their own problems. I hope I'm a walking sermon for them because I am trying to put what I tell them into action.

When I give advice nowadays, I'm not just mouthing things we learned to say in rabbinical school. Sometimes I believe I fell into the bad habit of performing my duties mechanically because they were part of my job. This awful illness has sparked me. It's almost as if I were living a new life as a rabbi. Maybe I had to struggle with this leukemia to be a more feeling person, so my ministry will be less automatic, more genuine.

My congregants notice the change in me. They say, "You put more meaning into the services." They tell me suddenly I'm listening much more to them. I've always been so hyper. One of my congregants told me the other day, "You're not in such a rush anymore. You were always the Running Rabbi—

it seemed you were trying to get away all the time. Now you're not frantically pursuing your next project, five miles ahead of us. You're waiting for us spiritually and in every way. You seem to be more open, and we can lean on you even more."

And he's right. I know I can't run away when people are telling me about their pain. I know what it is to be in deep trouble, so I can help others deal with theirs now. My congregants are always saying to me, "Well, Rabbi, you know . . ." They mean I know what it is to be critically ill and vulnerable. I know what it is to be faced with questions of life and death. I know what it is to suffer.

I remember reading Albert Schweitzer's book years ago, where he described how his own serious illness helped him identify more with his patients. He said something about a "fellowship of those who bear the mark of pain." It was such a beautiful phrase that it stuck with me. And there's a play by Sophocles about Philoctetes, a Greek soldier who was wounded on his way to the Trojan War. The other men left him on an island to die. The Greeks weren't defeating the Trojans so they went back to get Philoctetes because they heard he had developed a very accurate bow. With his bow they were able to conquer Troy, and the myth grew up of the "wounded healer": with our wounds we heal other people because of the moral triumph of suffering. Maybe I had to be "wounded" by this illness before I could try to heal others.

Now I don't let myself get away with anything other people might not even notice. Before my illness I made all the right condolence calls and said all the right things to someone in mourning, and I usually stopped at that. But now it's imperative with me that I not stop ministering to them, that I keep calling, keep checking on them, keep comforting them. It's a heavier burden, but it's the right thing to do. As my friend Stephanie Goldstein says, "The ticket has been filled in a little bit for you." You know what it is now to face death, and you know what it is when other people are facing tragedy. As long as you're going to call yourself a rabbi, you've got to keep working at it, helping and supporting people and expecting that of others.

It's something I live with now day in and day out with my congregants. We all teach and learn from each other: sometimes I don't know who is the rabbi and who the congregation. I've listened to one woman talk about her husband's stroke and depression so many times. She asks me to be strong for her, and I try to give her courage. I get strength from her too, because she has endured. Last year a congregant lost his job. I did what I could to help him relocate, but he's not back on his feet yet, and I'm still counseling him, trying to help him through his trauma.

My friend Paula and I have lunch together often and talk about how our illnesses have changed our lives. We go through cycles of helping each other. We are so bound up together in our struggles. She helps me cope with my leukemia, and I calm her fears that her Hodgkin's disease will recur and she'll have to face more radiation treatments.

Before this leukemia, sometimes I just did my duty. I would see somebody in a coffee shop or a supermarket and I would race by them. Jaffe had a style—I would wave to people, running past them in a hurry, give them a good feeling that I liked them. But now I stop and talk to them. It's been a real retraining. It's a realization of the way we should be. That is the godly thing to do, whatever religion you are. The way I try to see God is to perceive godliness in other human beings emerging in the special moments of life.

February 25, 1983

Today I met with my Newburgh Christian clergy friends, Father Fenlon and Reverend Henricksen, to record the interfaith radio program we do every two weeks. They always ask me how I'm doing, and they say, "See, Hirshel, now you have to place more trust in God." They are always saying, "Let God take over, Hirshel." I tell them we Jews believe we should be more active.

But now I think I'm beginning to come around to their view. I'm learning to relax a little and to rely more on God. What choice do I have now?

March 20, 1983

We just got back from the rabbinical convention in Los Angeles. I didn't want to go at first, didn't want to be that far away from my doctors, but Judi talked me into it. We had a great time.

The kids loved Disneyland. It was a perfect day when we went there. I sat in the bright sunshine and really relaxed. I forgot about my leukemia, and it seemed like things were really normal again. Rachel and Nina were able to see me as a father again instead of a sick person.

Ronnie drove us to the San Diego Zoo. He had to drag all our luggage for us because I didn't feel well enough to carry it. My wonderful little brother just couldn't do enough for us.

It is so important for me to travel, even though it's a big effort, because I just can't think about my illness all the time. You have to try to live a normal life even though it's always hanging over you and coloring your experiences.

Sometimes it's hard to get away from my illness. Little things constantly remind me of it. Like what happened a couple of weeks ago. It had been a really tough weekend. I didn't feel well. Somebody's uncle died, and I had another funeral the next day. I had to go to the cemetery, put together the evening services in the mourners' home. And there were two Bar Mitzvahs.

*I went to Burger King to take a break, and what happens?
I'm sort of half-listening to a group of teenagers talking at the
next table. Suddenly I realize they're talking about leukemia.
One kid is saying, "Oh, yes, that's when the white cells and
the immune system . . ." They're talking about what can be
done for it. It was uncanny.*

I couldn't finish my hamburger.

March 25, 1983

*The funniest thing happened at Greenhaven. I ordered
grape juice for the prisoners for the Passover seder in a few
days. The warden called me into his office. He was really
upset. He said, "Rabbi Jaffe, you're supposed to be bringing
grape juice in for the prisoners, not wine." I said, "I did order
grape juice." He said, "Well, the prisoners must have fer-
mented it because it's turned into wine."*

*The warden and I made a deal for next year. Next Passover
I won't bring the grape juice in so far ahead of time, and I'll
take responsibility for every bottle that comes in. The men will
have to drink it in front of me and sign for every bottle. I don't
know how that's going to work for the seder.*

*I think we Jews completely mystify the Greenhaven ad-
ministration. Last year one of the prisoners complained he
didn't have his tefillin. So I ordered him a set. When it arrived
he went to the security office to get it. The security man didn't
know tefillin is used for praying, and when the prisoner took
the tefillin out of the box the officer objected. He said it might
be a security risk. I guess he thought the prisoner could tie the
twelve-inch-long, thin leather straps together and hang himself, or attach the straps to a window and climb down to
escape!*

*Another terrible tragedy in our congregation. One of our
fine young families who worked with Jewish youth was visiting
relatives in Florida. They were driving in Miami yesterday and
a drunken driver hit them broadside. The father and seven-
year-old daughter were killed instantly. The mother and
twelve-year-old daughter, who were sitting on the other side of
the car, walked away with only scratches. A drunken driver
and a stolen car . . . it's almost unbelievable.*

*How many times I've had to deal with things like this! But
it's harder each time. These are the kinds of things we experience all the time as rabbis, and I should be used to it by now.
But I'm not. I'll never get used to it.*

*Here I am, I'm facing death, and I have to live with the fact
day in and day out that I may die slowly and painfully. But
death can hit anybody suddenly and totally unexpectedly, like
this terrible accident. Some people tell me that—to console
me, I guess. They say, "You don't have to be seriously ill to
confront death. It can happen anytime." They're right, of
course.*

*This made me put my own problems in perspective. Every-
body has his or her share of suffering. Suffering is universal.
But why did this accident have to happen? How can you make
sense out of a world where something like this happens? How
can I explain that to my congregants when I don't understand
it myself?*

*Sometimes we can't expect to find satisfying answers to
these agonizing questions. All of us, even rabbis, have to live
with our doubts and uncertainties. That's especially hard for
me since now I'm agonizing about my own fate. Once I may
have smugly thought I had some answers. But since my illness
I have known for sure that I don't. I'd like to be able to wave
a magic wand to find out why these wonderful people were*

killed in this dreadful accident and why I have this strange illness.

Why me?

Why anyone?

8

~~~~~

Finally the Rudin family is going to visit the Jaffes on Martha's Vineyard. . . .

The grueling drive from Manhattan takes six hours because of heavy traffic on Cape Cod. But we arrive at the Vineyard ferry slip at Wood's Hole an hour and a half early and position our car first in the automobile loading line. Anxious to stretch our legs, we lock the car and stroll around the dock.

Ten minutes before we're supposed to start driving the cars onto the ferry, we wander back to our car and discover I've locked the keys inside.

Everyone else in the automobile line is as panicked as we are—no one can drive onto the boat until we do because our car is blocking the entrance. Automobile reservations for the ferry to the island must be made months ahead of time. If these cars don't get onto this ferry they'll have to stay at Wood's Hole because there will be no room for them on the other boats. There are only about eight ferries a day, with hundreds of cars and trucks fighting for space, and a huge standby list. Everyone in our line is eager to get to the Vineyard and enjoy the long Memorial Day weekend.

The driver of the car behind us opens her trunk and produces a wire clothing hanger. She and I take turns easing the hanger through a tiny space at the top of our front window and trying to pull the door lock up with the hanger's hook.

It's time to load the cars onto the ferry, and we still haven't opened the car door with the hanger. The drivers in the cars behind us start to honk their horns. The men in charge of loading the cars onto the ferry give us dirty looks. Marcia is nagging me; Eve and Jennifer are whining. Everyone is watching us. Perspiration dribbles down my back.

Finally the woman with the hanger succeeds in jiggling the lock up, and we open the door and pile into our car quickly. Everyone in the line cheers as we drive up the gangplank and onto the boat.

After we arrive at the Jaffes' house and unload the car, I take the drink Judi made for me out to the deck, put my feet up on the railing, and for the first time that day just relax.

The view from the Jaffes' deck is beautiful. The white sands of South Beach on the Atlantic Ocean stretch as far as the eye can see, and the surf pounds the shore in a regular, soothing rhythm. In the distance I spot Hirshel jogging slowly with Rachel and Nina and their big old English sheepdog named Monday. It is so good to see my friend running again. I know how much it means to him. I haven't seen Hirshel since last December. He looks much better than he did then. It's nearly a year since his leukemia was diagnosed. Even from this distance I can see he has put on some badly needed weight and that he has good color.

Hirshel sees me sitting up here on the deck and waves. Rachel and Nina run off to find our children. "Let's take a walk on the beach," he calls out to me. "It's so beautiful in the late afternoon. We won't be having dinner for a while."

I take off my sneakers and hot, sweaty socks and leave

them on the deck. The tide is going out, and the sand feels cool under my bare feet.

"It's great to see you running again, Hirshel."

"I'm feeling pretty good, Jim. I've adjusted to having less energy because of my lower blood count. I go in for blood tests more often now. I just had one at the Martha's Vineyard Hospital. I'm down to 100,000 platelets. Normal range is 185,000 to 350,000, so you can see my count is getting lower all the time. My leukemia might not be headed for the long remission the specialist in Chicago predicted. We have to watch it constantly. But I'm working as much as I can. My biggest fear is that someday I'll be too sick to work."

"I know what you're scared of. I know how important working is to you. But, Hirshel, maybe it would be better for you now if you weren't a rabbi. In a strange way, your work, your particular work as a rabbi, constantly reminds you of your own troubles because as rabbis we're never very far away from suffering and illness and death. You can't just excuse yourself from the case, as a lawyer can. If you were an accountant, you could go back to keeping books, bury yourself in numbers, and get pleasure from them, and forget about yourself. But ironically, immersing yourself in *your* job has the opposite effect."

"That's very true, Jim. After I got home from the hospital last fall, a friend of mine said, 'Hirshel, you're going to be raw, you're going to be vulnerable, don't do funerals for a while. So for a few weeks I didn't. Until those people died in the fire and left two children. I felt I had to do their funeral, no matter how difficult it was for me. But I wouldn't change professions now. Being a rabbi does make it harder to forget my illness, but it has advantages too. It enables me to channel my experience into helping other people. I can even pray with them now, which I never did before."

103

"Do you really pray now, Hirshel?"

"Well, the prayers in the liturgy are more real for me now. There were times before my illness when I was stale. Sometimes I was repeating the prayers like a robot, the same prayers over and over again for twenty years, not much intensity except on rare occasions.

"You know, Jim, it's hard to get yourself into a prayer when you're officiating. You're absorbed too much with running the services—will the choir come in on time at the right place, and is the Torah open to the right portion for the week, are we hitting every cue just right? I still have to worry about all those details, but now before services I go into my study and open the prayer book and read it and really think about what the prayers say. I never did that before. Now I pray privately before I go out onto the pulpit, and sometimes I make up my own prayers at different times during the day.

"I'll be alone in the car, thinking about Judi and the children and my struggle, and I'll voice my thoughts out loud in a prayerful way, usually something like, 'God, give me the strength,' or 'God, let me keep up my spirits.' I pray I can have many more moments with my family and my friends, times like this—walking on this beautiful beach that I love with you, one of my oldest friends. I know how precious these times are. I do it when people ask how I'm getting along. My answers have become prayers now. Sometimes my funeral eulogies or my sermons become prayers. Well, maybe they're not prayers, they're more like affirmations or statements."

"Those are prayers, Hirshel. If you're thinking about your family and your life, that's praying."

"And I recite Psalm 121: 'I lift up my eyes to the mountains from whence cometh my help.' I've said that so many times at services and funerals it's almost a part of me. It has a special meaning for me now. I'm asking

God to help me get up the mountain I'm climbing because I'm no longer the Hirshel Jaffe who could run up the ski lift in Vail, Colorado, or halfway up Pike's Peak, which I did once on a dare. Now God is helping me up the mountain. Or put it this way—I pray for the strength and courage to make it up.

"Before my illness I thought, 'What do I have to pray for? I have the physical strength and courage.' But now I'm praying for another kind of courage, another kind of strength, spiritual stamina for a different kind of climb. Not necessarily to make it up to the top of the mountain, but just so I won't fall down again. We're all like climbers, trying to conquer life's precipices."

"You keep using the mountain-climbing image, Hirshel, and I don't know exactly what you mean."

"It means to not let myself despair. To keep up my spirits. To have hope. Not giving up my work, my family . . . my life. I guess it means making the best of my situation, making the most out of life. To be positive and not fall prey to depression. You remember, Jim, I nearly gave up before I had my second operation last summer? I wasn't prepared for that terrible experience in the hospital. I'd never been tested, and I lost hope too soon."

"Well, you had a right to be depressed. Things did look pretty bad there for a while, Hirshel. I even prayed for you myself. But I am never sure God is listening."

"I'm not either. I don't think God is up there pulling strings and saying, 'Hirshel will get better, Hirshel won't get better.' Yet somehow I've learned to trust my fate more to God. God is entering the picture more now.

"It's not that He'll intervene directly or pull off a miracle. But God isn't so abstract for me anymore. I use the word 'God' and it means more to me. I'm saying, 'I can't do it all on my own, so You take over a little bit, God.' For the first time I'm seeing God as a loving, caring parent you place your burdens on. Maybe that's an unsophisticated concept of God for a rabbi who has studied theology, but that's how I feel. Gee, Jim, it's starting to get late. We'd better turn around and head back to the house."

The sun, so big on the horizon over the ocean, is beginning to set. The colors in the sky are vivid and beautiful. The beach is nearly empty now, and it is very peaceful. We turn around and retrace our footsteps in the sand.

"You remember, Jim, in rabbinical school how we'd treat the subject of God lightly. We were so familiar with the concept. Deep down I was self-absorbed, selfish, narcissistic, and I was saying, 'What do I need God for? I am God.' Now for the first time I'm realizing I'm not. So in that sense I'm saying let God take over, I can't do it all myself. Before, I always felt I had to explain everything verbally and rationally. I don't think so anymore. Now it's enough for me to just feel it with my heart."

"I don't think we talked very much about God in rabbinical school, not about God in a personal sense," I say.

"No. I didn't become a rabbi because I felt God wanted me to, did you, Jim? No, for me it was more a desire to transmit our heritage. The Jewish ideas were so important in my family, since my father was a Jewish educator. I wanted to pass them on to the next generation. I got a real kick out of teaching religious school while I was in college, and I took courses at Hebrew Union College to help me with my teaching. One day the rabbi at the synagogue where I taught, a distinguished-looking man with white hair, said to me, 'Jaffe, you would make a good rabbi.' That started me thinking about it. My parents were very pleasantly surprised.

"Then there was the whole social justice thing. I was looking around for something meaningful to do. I attended business school for a while, you know, and I toyed around with the idea of becoming a labor arbitrator—a sort of 'arbitrator of people,' I guess. Those were the days of the civil rights struggle and other causes. I always had a strong moral conscience. My friends called me the moral bug. My fraternity at City College was the first one on campus to integrate blacks into it. I was so impressed by Judaism's prophetic tradition and what it offered the world."

"We all wanted to change the world in those days, Hirshel. Most Reform rabbis wanted to be social reformers. I became a rabbi primarily to help the Jewish people survive, but I spoke out on social issues too. I marched for civil rights and went to jail in Mississippi with other rabbis and Protestant ministers. That was scary—they were shooting 'outside agitators' down there then. It's different now. Rabbinical students and the young reform rabbis today are still interested in social justice, but they're more spiritually oriented, more traditional and religious than we are."

"But I'm moving in that direction now, Jim. Since my illness I've become more open to possibilities about God and about prayer and afterlife, all those things. I was more buttoned down before. Of course, I feel sheepish and slightly guilty, because I had to get sick before I took these concepts more seriously. I used to preach to my congregants—I'd say, 'God isn't just for bad times, He's for good times too.' But I didn't follow my own advice. I guess that's only human—you don't think you need God until you run into trouble. But as a rabbi I shouldn't have waited until I felt helpless to acknowledge my need for God.

"Now I'm more willing to look at the Jewish tradition on its own terms. Like the Book of Life we talk about at Rosh Hashana. I still don't believe in it literally, but I was deeply moved by it during the last High Holidays because of my illness. The Book of Life idea wasn't any more theologically coherent than before, but it was more emotionally meaningful. I was thinking, 'I've made it so far, but what will happen in the future?' It evoked all that for me. The theology doesn't have to be that literal.

"I'm turning to the Jewish tradition more because it's amazingly right. It teaches us to choose life. Not to despair. We're a people of hope. The idea of death doesn't scare me so much anymore, Jim. I've been grappling so much with life and death, and that schools you. Before I got sick, living forever was almost like proving my endurance, setting another record, finishing a marathon. But it's not a question of that now, I've come to terms with that. My blood counts are going down, and it might be just a matter of time before my remission ends. Maybe I'm learning to accept the inevitable."

"Does Judaism help you accept your illness? As a rabbi, you've quoted the Bible and the Talmud to people who are ill, or to their families. Do those passages help you now?"

"Yes, they do help. But words aren't enough."

"Our friend Ronnie Sobel told me an interesting story, Hirshel. When a prominent minister's son was killed in an automobile accident, Ronnie wrote him a condolence note. The minister never answered the letter, but later he said, 'Rabbi Sobel, your note was the only one that comforted me. All the other clergy who wrote to me quoted from Scripture. I know all those passages. I know Scripture better than anybody else. You were the only one who didn't throw Bible verses at me, and I appreciated it.' "

"It's true, Jim, People want to hear more than Bible quotes. Words and formulas alone can't bring enough comfort."

"So what does help, Hirshel? What helps *you?*"

"The real comfort comes when you know that other people care about you. You know, Jim, we only have each other in this life. We only have other people. Do you remember that Hassidic story about the burning embers we learned in rabbinical school? A Hassid is complaining to his rebbe that he is depressed. He feels alone, there is illness and a business setback in his family, and he is afraid God doesn't care about him. They are sitting in front of the fire, talking, and the fire is just about to go out. There are only scattered embers in the fireplace. The rebbe takes the poker and stokes the embers into a heap. There is a burst of flame and new warmth from the fire.

" 'You see?' the rebbe says to his student. 'Do you see what happened when I gathered the embers closer together? The fire came back to life. When the coals are separated from each other, there is little heat. But when they are close to each other, they get warmth from each other and the fire is renewed. It's the same with people. When we are alone and separated or disconnected from each other our spirit is in danger of dying out. But when we huddle together, we get warmth and comfort from one another, and hope is renewed.' "

"On his deathbed the Baal Shem Tov said something like 'Take hold one with the other.' He meant that we shouldn't be separate."

"Well, Jim, that's the kind of warmth I am getting from my family and friends through all this. From my non-Jewish friends too, like our neighbors in Newburgh. You always wonder what these people really think of Jews, of my being a rabbi. But they've really supported me.

"You know, since this illness I've been struck by the universality of religion and of God. The specific theology isn't as important as the fact that we're all children of God. That's one reason I admire you so much, because you're in the field of interfaith relations. That's always been very crucial to me. I've worked hard at interreligious understanding in Newburgh, and it hasn't always been easy. Since my illness I've been speaking in more universal terms than ever before. Jim, this is not a *Jewish* leukemia. You shouldn't only help Jews. Why does religion have to be so parochial?

"This has been a real learning experience for me. I know that sounds strange. Some people say God allows us to suffer so we can learn from it. I think I'm beginning to agree with that. It's a tough way to learn, but look, Jim, I've got the disease. It's a fact. Since I'm stuck with it, I might as well try to meet the challenge. I can make it a positive experience, try to grow as a person instead of just complaining. Instead of wondering, 'Why me, why did this happen to me?' you can say, 'I've got the disease, now what can I do with it?' You have to look forward, not backward. Life isn't fair, but you can't give up. You have to ask, 'What am I going to do about this lack of fairness?' "

"Ronnie Sobel said it beautifully. He said to me once, 'It's whether you use the painful experience for enrichment or for embitterment. It's whether you feel more love than you might have. It's whether you have more understanding than you might have.' "

"Yes, Jim, I do think my life is more enriched. I do feel more love and understanding than I did before all this happened. Maybe that's the reason for it, the meaning in it I've been looking for. But I don't want to kid you—I'm bitter and angry too. You asked me last August when I first found out about my leukemia if I was angry. I think I said, 'No.' Well, I've changed my mind. Sometimes I am. I'm damned angry at what I've gone through. I'm angry when I think about what lies ahead for me and for my family. I'm angry because I don't think we deserve it. . . . Oh, Jim, I can see Judi waving us in from the deck. Dinner must be ready."

We speed up our steps and walk quickly back the remaining length of the beach to the Jaffes' house.

Suddenly I realize how hungry I am.

9

~~~

W*e just got back from Eve Rudin's Bat Mitzvah. God,
how do these kids grow up so fast? I'm so glad I went.
We almost didn't go because I wasn't feeling well this morning, and it's a long drive into New York City.*

*Eve chanted her Torah portion beautifully. A lot of my old
rabbi friends were there. It was good to see everybody again.*

*Only seven more months until Rachel's Bat Mitzvah in
April! I hope I make it. I hope I'll be well enough to be able
to enjoy it. People are always saying, "Just let me live until my
grandson's Bar Mitzvah," or "Just let me see my grandchild's
wedding." Well, now I'm saying that. That's a new goal I've
set for myself, and it keeps me going because I yearn so badly
to share in that beautiful day.*

*September 27, 1983
Sukkot*

What a funny scene today . . .

*A group of Lubavicher Hassidim from Brooklyn comes into
Greenhaven regularly as volunteers to visit the prisoners. They
asked if they could bring a "Sukkahmobile" into the prison.
I brought it up to the warden and he said it would be OK.*

113

So today about twenty Hassidim drive into the prison yard with their flatbed truck. The prison guards are looking under the truck and searching it, making sure they're not smuggling anything into the prison with it. Well, the Hassidim start dancing and juggling and doing acrobatics to entertain the prisoners.

The black and Puerto Rican prisoners and the guards are taking in the scene, staring at these guys in their black suits and their beards and their long sideburns looking like people out of another century. I don't think they could believe what they were seeing. The Hassidim led all the prisoners in a cheer, "We want Messiah now." I heard one of the prisoners watching ask, "Who's Messiahnow?" Then the Hassidim bring out all the delicious food—noodle kugel and honey cakes and nuts and raisins—and the Jewish guys are stuffing it in their pockets to take back to their cells.

October 10, 1983

I went apple picking with Judi and the girls and some friends for the second year in a row. We go to a place about ten miles from Newburgh called Apple Valley. You get on little trucks and they take you into the orchards.

Our friends brought crackers and cheese and wine and spread out a blanket. Judi and Rachel and Nina knocked the apples down with long poles while I rested on the blanket. Everybody took pictures. It was such a gorgeous day. I sat under a tree watching them, and it was a "normal" day. I was hardly thinking about my leukemia at all.

It was just beautiful.

Maybe you really do have to experience bad things like my illness in order to appreciate the good things in life. Maybe we do need the contrast. I know since I got sick I've relished the simple, everyday things with my family and friends. I was

114

always jumpy, anxious to rush on to the next activity. Now I can relax and savor the present.

November 5, 1983

This illness has taught me the real meaning of the rabbinate. The most important thing is not who can be the best scholar. I remember in rabbinical school I was always winning contests for Hebrew proficiency or grammar. The other guys were married, but all I ever did was study. I always put so much value on intellectual achievement. My whole family does. But now I've moved away from the cerebral. It's who can best minister to people's needs that really matters. It's who can touch people, who can comfort people.

We weren't properly prepared for pastoral work in rabbinical school. Our professors lived in an ivory tower. They had a cynical view of congregational life. They wanted us to be scholars. We got emotional about the tradition and what the rabbis said twenty centuries ago, and there were some very moving stories, but there was nothing about today. *We didn't intern at hospitals or consult with psychiatrists or train with senior rabbis in the field. This is changing in seminaries now.*

Some of this you just can't learn in school—it has to come from long experience. I've learned in my twenty years as a rabbi and especially since this illness that God wants heart. There's a Hebrew expression, Rachmana liba baey—*"God wants heart." I think the word* rachmanis *is the* key word in *Judaism. More important than any theology or system of thought is the caring, the compassion, the loving, the* rachmanis. *Judi always nags me about this. She'll say, "Hirshel, you didn't really touch that boy in the Bar Mitzvah today. You didn't really mean it."*

I'm thinking about this tonight because this afternoon I had

115

a fight with an older rabbi in a nearby community. He had castigated a woman for not following Jewish law, and he hurt her feelings. She came to me and related her story. So today I went back to this rabbi who is rooted so rigidly in the tradition and I said to him, "Don't you know the teaching in our Talmud, Rachmana liba baey? That over and above what is theologically accurate or what is proper according to the law, what is just, God wants compassion, He wants feeling, He wants heart?"

I've tried to make my congregants aware of rachmanis too. When I first came back from the hospital last year, I challenged everyone in the congregation. That was my first message to the board of trustees when I went back to work. I made them promise they would give the same comfort to everyone else that they gave to me. We formed a caring committee and we have pins with little people holding hands on them. The committee organizes minyans and visits people in nursing homes and hospitals, and they visit the handicapped. They take the retarded to services at our temple.

November 20, 1983

My blood counts are still going down. Yesterday when I drove to Greenhaven Prison I felt so weak I got out of my car in the parking lot very slowly. I leaned on it for a minute to rest before I started the long walk to my chaplaincy office.

When I got to the office, my telephone was ringing. It was the prison infirmary. The nurse asked, "Are you all right, Rabbi Jaffe?" I said, "Yes, why?" She said, "One of the prison guards on the wall saw you get out of your car very carefully and walk slowly. He said in all the years you've been coming here he has never seen you walk so slowly. He was concerned and he telephoned me and asked me to check on you."

I said to the nurse, "I see even a prison has heart."

Today in our temple lobby a woman in my congregation asked Judi where she has been. The woman said, "We haven't seen you at services for so long, since the High Holidays." Judi said, "Well, I'll tell you." Right in front of everyone Judi says, "You see, I'm fooling around, and Friday night is the only night I'm sure where Hirshel is going to be."

When I heard that I couldn't believe it!

Years ago when we were in Dallas Judi was working in the Parkland Hospital trauma unit. One of the Sisterhood members asked her why she wasn't coming to the next luncheon. Judi said to her, "What if your child was in the trauma unit and the nurse, Mrs. Jaffe, couldn't take care of it because she was at the Sisterhood lunch?"

My congregants love Judi, and she can get away with anything because she is so outrageous, she's such a blunt and honest person. She disarms people. Judi's really tough. She saw her father dying for a long time when she was young, and I think that kept her from having illusions about life. This realism is sustaining her now. That and faith in God.

Judi's faith in God has always been much more direct than mine. She always says, "Why are you telling me all this silly theology, Hirshel? Just believe." Judi has never questioned God. I have never heard her say a cynical word about God. About people, yes, but never about God.

That really surprises people. They would never think Judi believes in God that strongly because of her tough exterior and her humor. And it surprises me too because she's never exactly enjoyed being a rabbi's wife. It's very hard to be married to someone in the clergy, and she hates having a functionary role imposed on her, because she insists on being herself. She doesn't come to services very often. When she does it isn't for show, and she slips unobtrusively into the back row of the sanctuary.

But Judi's not against genuine religion. Sometimes she'll point out an ultra-Orthodox family and say, "See, Hirshel, that's real religion." It's not that Judi and I think being Orthodox is the only way to be genuinely religious or genuinely Jewish. But she wants to incorporate the passion and commitment the Orthodox so often have into our religious lives.

Maybe some of Judi's kind of faith is rubbing off on me.

December 23, 1983

Last night at a temple board meeting one of the older board members said something I disagreed with. Immediately I spoke out. I wouldn't have done that before my illness. I would have kept my feelings to myself, accommodated. I guess by suffering and becoming so human and being forced to fight for my life I've gotten to be more of a fighter in general. That helps you in every phase of life.

That's just one of the things I've learned from this whole experience.

I've learned you shouldn't feel cursed if you have a disease with a foul name. Don't think of yourself as worth less or worthless because you've been stricken. People tend to blame themselves for their misfortune. They think they must have done something wrong, and they feel guilty if they're too sick to do anything.

Tell the people you love how you feel about them while you still have the chance.

Be kind to yourself. Hug yourself if you can't find anybody to hug you. When you have an illness, you learn all of a sudden that you have to pay attention to yourself. You have to become more selfish.

You have to admit to yourself that you're not Superman. You can't do the impossible, and you can't do everything. You can't have complete control over your fate. You have to let go and relinquish some control. There's a saying—"To let go is to gain control." Well, that's been very hard for me. I've had to learn how to do it. And you have to stop spinning your wheels and trying to please everybody. You can't be responsible for everybody anymore.

I'm learning to say no to people. You can't fritter your life away and let somebody else tell you how to live. You shouldn't let your doctors determine your entire fate. Don't lose your life because you're afraid of them. I said to my doctor once, "Hey, it's my body, it's me that has the cancer." And of course he had to say, "You're right."

Don't lament the past and fill yourself with regrets. Don't keep thinking, "I should have gone to another doctor," or "Why didn't they spot my illness sooner?" or "There must be something else we should be doing." You just get depressed, and it's counterproductive.

Don't hide your illness from people. Be frank. And don't let other people try to duck it or ignore it and pretend everything's OK or talk around it because they're uncomfortable. Some people actually avoid me because cancer frightens them. A few of my friends are having a tough time phoning or visiting because they can't deal with my illness.

Take the help other people can give you. Sometimes it's just moral support. Or maybe they'll drive you somewhere or run an errand or make a phone call or help you carry a package. One of my congregants is always offering to read some of the prayers in Shabbat services. It's a little thing, but it does lighten my load, and it makes him feel better too. You have to learn it's not a sign of weakness to let other people do what they can to make things easier for you.

I let my daughters help me now. I'm more accepting of the love they offer me when they know I'm down. Sometimes Nina will give me a little hug or a pat on the shoulder. Rachel will ask me if I want a blanket when I lie down to rest. These are little things, but it's their way of showing they love me.

119

I'm more frank with my daughters now. I don't avoid them when I come home after having my blood tested, and I tell them what the doctors say. I think my new openness about my disease is helping them cope, although sometimes I feel guilty about overloading their young lives with the weight of my illness. But being dishonest and trying to hide things from them just hurts them and makes them feel left out. You can't fool kids. They're smart and they always sense what's going on.

Now I'm much more definite with my children and with my life in general. I don't sit around wondering if maybe we'll do this or maybe we'll do that or we'll do it when we have the money or when I'm in the mood. When something comes to me I do it. Now the kids know when Daddy says, "This is the time," we do it. Judi has been taken aback a few times, but I think she likes that kind of assertiveness from me.

I decide to call Hirshel at his synagogue to wish him a happy New Year.

Hirshel and I like to kid each other on the phone with our fake voices. Once when we were on Martha's Vineyard together some years ago, I was anxiously waiting for my entry visa to come through from the Soviet Union so I could lead an interreligious delegation to the USSR. Hirshel called our cottage and whispered in an authentic-sounding Russian accent, "Rabbi Rudin, this is the Soviet embassy. Your visa has been denied."

Since then I have been trying to outdo him. So today when I phone the synagogue I tell Hirshel's secretary I'm from the Internal Revenue Service and I want to audit Rabbi Jaffe's taxes. I hear panic in her voice as she puts me on hold, running into Hirshel's office, I assume, to give him the bad news.

Hirshel comes on the phone and apprehensively says, "Hello?"

"Rabbi Jaffe, your papers are not in order, and ve vant to audit your income taxes," I say in my best Eastern European accent.

"Jim, is that you?"

"I can never fool you anymore. I just wanted to wish you and Judi a happy New Year."

"Thank you, same to you. Well, I made it to 1984. I'm trying to keep my spirits up because I know that's so important now. I have my good and bad days. But my counts are still going down slowly. And I have this irritating dry cough."

Hirshel's voice often takes on a self-pitying tone these days. It annoys me, and today I can't restrain myself.

"Hirshel," I snap, "I hope you won't take this the wrong way, but it seems to me you sometimes let your illness make you into the Suffering Servant. You know, Isaiah 53: 'A man of pains and acquainted with disease . . . he carries our diseases and pains,' or something like that. Don't you think you're sort of playing a role? Favoring your illness as someone would favor an injured leg?"

Hirshel is silent. I realize I've hurt his feelings, and suddenly I feel guilty. Who am I to scold my friend for feeling sorry for himself? I'm perfectly healthy. You've got a lot of nerve, Jim, I berate myself.

"Well, Jim, you know I have been through a lot!" Hirshel says angrily. He pauses. "But I guess you're right. I do tend to dramatize things."

"I'm sorry I said that, Hirshel. But honestly, sometimes it's hard to be patient with you."

"I know. Judi tells me that all the time. I do use my illness as a mental crutch when I'm feeling down. I'm embarrassed and ashamed when I catch myself doing it.

121

Judi checks me, and the children sense it too. They'll say, 'Is Daddy acting sick again?' and I can tell they're disgusted with me. They want me to be normal, and they're right. I'm conscious of the tendency to play the martyr, but I think I'm overcoming it now. It's important to just step back and observe yourself once in a while.

"It's interesting, Jim, even though you get sick and your life changes so much, you're no different than you were before. You're still the same person with all the same faults. You think you'll change and become a better person, but you don't."

"People don't really change. Hirshel, are you trying to become a saint?"

"Maybe I am."

"Don't. Just be yourself. You have enough to cope with."

I want to apologize to Hirshel again for rebuking him, and I want to tell my friend that we all love him just the way he is. But I have trouble expressing my feelings.

For the rest of the day I'm angry at myself for losing my temper with Hirshel. What kind of friend are you, I keep reproaching myself. You're supposed to be supporting Hirshel, not criticizing him. I feel rotten. Marcia tries to make me feel better. "You're only human, Jim," she tells me. But still I feel I am failing Hirshel. Just when he needs me most.

January 16, 1984

Rachel is doing fantastically with her ice skating. She just can't get enough of it.

Today I drove her to her lesson. It was wonderful to watch her pirouetting on the ice in her pretty skating dress. She's so graceful. I enjoy my children so much. Especially now, when

I know I might not have much time left with them, I treasure every minute we can share. Since I've gotten leukemia I "number my days," as the Bible tells us. I've come to cherish my limited time on earth.

I can't imagine my life without Rachel and Nina. For Jews it's a Mitzvah to have children. We're commanded to "be fruitful and multiply." We're always worried about preserving our existence, since the Jewish population is dwindling. But that's not the only reason for having them. I agree with what the Jewish tradition says about children: they are a blessing and a joy.

February 3, 1984

I'm learning to laugh at myself more. I guess it's "gallows humor."

Today I found some shoes I liked and I bought two pairs, black and brown. I said to myself, "Hirshel, will you get enough use out of them?" And once when Nina was opening up a can of Nine Lives cat food, she read the label out loud and said, "Here, Daddy, you could use some of this."

I've learned to laugh not only at trivial things, but at serious and even horrendous things. My ability to laugh has grown more and more as my health problems get tougher.

You have to laugh. It's the only way to survive.

February 15, 1984

Our wonderful dog, Monday, died. I feel like I've lost one of my children! We had her for thirteen years. She was so big and furry and lovable.

I named a baby in our congregation today too. One death, one birth. The life cycle goes on. . . .

March 4, 1984

Jim phoned me today. It's the tenth anniversary of his brother's death. . . .

Yesterday one of the Hassidic Lubavicher rabbis from Brooklyn came into my office at Greenhaven Prison and said, "Let me have your Hebrew name. I'm going to see the rebbe in three weeks. He's a very busy man, but I'm going to give him your name and he'll recite a prayer for you." I could tell he believed it. I was cynical, because I don't believe that kind of remote incantation is going to help me.

But I was touched anyway because it meant he cared about me. It's not the recitation of your name but the concern of the person that helps you. The efficacy lies not in the prayer but in who is saying it.

March 28, 1984
My 48th birthday!

This morning before I opened my birthday cards and gifts on the kitchen table, I jokingly asked Judi and the girls, "Do you know what Daddy wants for his birthday?" Right out of the blue Rachel said, "A cure?" We all laughed.

But her spontaneous remark made me realize how close to the surface Rachel's thoughts and fears about me are. I sometimes forget how much this is on my daughters' minds. Especially Rachel, who is so busy with her hair and her makeup and her girl friends and the pictures of rock stars taped up on her bedroom walls. And now she's busy practicing her Hebrew chanting, preparing for her Bat Mitzvah next month. She appears to be leading the life of a normal adolescent. But I can see this must be affecting her deeply.

Nina expresses her feelings more directly. Tonight Judi told me that Nina asked her this morning after I opened my gifts,

124

"Is Daddy going to die?"—the same question she asked in the pathology lab when they discovered my leukemia.

I guess she never gets that out of her thoughts. Somehow, even without my telling her, she always senses when I'm going to the doctor to have my blood checked. She says, "Let's find the best doctor in the world for you, Daddy." When I went out to see the hairy-cell leukemia specialist in Chicago last October, I told Nina I had been to a really big expert, and she asked, "Does he know you by heart, Daddy?" I think that's remarkable sensitivity for an eleven-year-old.

But dammit, why do my kids have to go through this? Why can't they just have the usual teenage worries? Why do they have to wonder if their daddy's going to die?

When they went back to school after my spleenectomy, Rachel's teacher asked her class to write an essay on "What I did during my summer vacation." Rachel wrote, "I went to camp. I had a wonderful time. My daddy got leukemia." The teacher telephoned Judi. She was terribly upset.

I don't want Rachel's teachers pitying her. I don't want my girls singled out. It's bad enough going through life as a rabbi's daughter. I just want them to be normal. I don't want my girls to have this pain. Life is hard enough without having to cope with something like this at their age.

Damn! Damn! Damn!

I told Jim once we don't curse God, but sometimes I can't help it. It all seems so unfair.

For the thousandth time I ask, "Why!?"

April 3, 1984

I've done some hilarious weddings in my lifetime, but this one has to take the cake. No pun intended.

The wedding was up at Lake Mohonk, a beautiful glacial lake near New Paltz, New York, about twenty miles from

125

Newburgh. *Everything had a Spanish motif—the women were all dressed in Spanish costumes.*

The ceremony took place on some rocks that hung over a glacier. All the old people were having trouble trying to climb out onto the rocks. It was very cold and windy. During the ceremony I kept trying to keep from falling off the rock in all the wind. I was the closest person to the water. It was about a five-hundred-foot drop to the water.

The couple requested that as part of the wedding ceremony I read from Kahlil Gibran's The Prophet. *But unfortunately about a week ago I read a parody of his poetry called* The Profit, *and as I was reading* The Prophet *in the ceremony I kept thinking of the parody. Between that and trying to keep from falling off the rock into the water, I could barely keep a straight face.*

It was even funnier than the wedding I did a couple of years ago when they had just watered the flowers decorating the canopy and the water started dripping all over me and the bride and groom as I was reading the ceremony.

April 13, 1984

While Judi was reading the Vineyard Gazette, *she saw that someone on Martha's Vineyard was selling golden retriever puppies born on March twenty-eighth. March twenty-eighth is my birthday, and we saw a good omen in that. We've wanted a new dog since Monday died, so we went up to the Vineyard and bought one of the puppies.*

She is a little darling. The girls named her Lexi, short for Alexis. I love this dog. She's so full of life, so irrepressible.

She sits in the front seat of the jeep when I drive and puts her head on my shoulder, and she likes to sit on my lap. It's so important to have something to cuddle when you're sick.

Lexi came with me today to watch Nina ride in a horse

show. Nina won another red ribbon to add to her collection. She is a wonderful horsewoman, and she looks great on a horse, her little slim body so erect.

She makes me so proud.

10

〜〜〜

I decide to telephone Hirshel to make arrangements about my part in Rachel's Bat Mitzvah. A long time ago I promised my friend I would officiate at his daughter's Sabbath morning Bat Mitzvah service. But his voice sounds strained and subdued, and I ask him what's the matter.

"I just went back and forth to Albany today, Jim. I'm very tired. And I got some bad news. You know, things have been going pretty well. Even though my platelet count has been low, I've been able to function. But about a week ago when I was visiting a nursing home I suddenly felt very weak and shook up and I was trembling. Then last Friday night during services I could hardly lift the Torah over my head. And my cough's getting worse. So I called my hematologist and pushed up the date for my checkup.

"He tested my blood as usual, but his face fell when he got the results. I have only 75,000 platelets, and I'm getting anemic. When I went out to see the specialist in Chicago last October, he told me not to worry until my blood count goes down to 90,000. He said I should telephone him then. And here it is only 75,000. In two months I've dropped from 100,000 to 75,000—25 percent of my platelets! And my white cells are acting funny.

"My hematologist said flatly, 'It's time you start treatment.' He suggested I go to Albany to see a specialist he knows there. Judi drove me there today. The specialist examined me and looked over my records and took his own blood tests. Then he said, 'Well, Rabbi, it looks like your disease has become active. We should begin treatment. We don't have that much of a margin to wait, or the treatment won't avail us.'

"That was a fancy way of saying, 'Or it will be too late.' My heart sank at the bad news. But I was relieved that there's some sort of active treatment available, and I was glad he was being so honest with me. He gave me the parameters of my situation and discussed the various therapy options and said that I have to make the choice myself. He let me be the person to make the decision. Not all the doctors do that. Sometimes they leave you completely out of it.

"He suggested I take leukeran, a new form of oral chemotherapy. It's the most benign chemotherapy around. 'Least toxic' is the phrase he used. The doctors have always told me stronger chemotherapy doesn't help hairy-cell leukemia and might only hurt me. If this leukeran doesn't work and my blood counts don't start to go back up, we'll stop it at the end of six months and I'll begin to take a drug called interferon. I phoned the specialist in Chicago, and he agreed with these steps. He'll take me into his interferon program there."

"Isn't interferon still an experimental drug?" I ask.

"Yes. And it can have bad side effects. No one knows exactly what they'll be because they're different for everybody. Some people get high fevers and chills. You can lose your appetite and get listless. But it seems to be the only choice I have now besides the leukeran. And they say it's showing a lot of promise with my disease. I'll take two leukeran pills a day for six months. They don't have terrible side effects like stronger chemotherapy does."

I know all about those side effects. I don't want to remind Hirshel that my brother, Bert, suffered terribly from them.

"However, the doctor said the leukeran is a two-edged sword," Hirshel continues. "While it kills the cancer cells in my bone marrow, it could suppress my normal cells too and I could get an infection or bleeding. He told me I probably won't notice anything for the first two or three months, but I might run into trouble in the third month. He said, 'We might have to save you in the third month.' That was scary. But if I can get through that rough period, the leukeran might help me in the long run. Look, Jim, I don't want to worry you. Please don't breathe a word of this to anybody at the Bat Mitzvah, especially my family. I don't want to ruin the happy day for them."

"Hirshel, are you going to take the leukeran?"

"Of course. There's no question in my mind. If I didn't take it, I would be committing suicide."

Slowly I hang up the phone. "So now it begins," I think. How many times have I heard these terrifying words, "If I didn't take the treatment, I would be committing suicide"? In nearly every cancer case it often comes down to that phrase or one similar to it. For Hirshel it is a kind of personal continental divide: since his spleenectomy, the disease has been in remission, He has had no medication, radiation, or other major treatments. But with this transition to drug therapy, from now on everything will be very different for him.

Right now Hirshel has the leukeran option, and that sounds hopeful. But what if the pills have bad side effects? Can any chemotherapy be really "benign"? He will be putting powerful drugs into his body. And what if the leukeran doesn't work and Hirshel has to turn to interferon? Will the benefits he gets from this radical, experimental treatment be worth the bad side effects he might suffer?

After the interferon, what? A bone marrow transplant? The physicians told Hirshel that wouldn't work, and I know it is a dangerous and extremely painful procedure. My family considered it for Bert when nothing else was stopping his Hodgkin's disease. My brother's physicians advised us not to put him through the ordeal.

What is ahead for Hirshel Jaffe? Will he opt to continue treating his cancer? These are the haunting questions now.

An increasing number of cancer patients are refusing all chemotherapy and radiation therapies because they see the agony and suffering these procedures often bring. Some highly invasive treatments extend life for only a brief time at best. "Why," they argue, "should I undergo such horrendous therapy for only a slightly longer life?"

Should we preserve and extend life in spite of intense pain and suffering? Is a life wracked with incurable cancer better than no life at all? Isn't a person's right to die as important as the right to live?

I remember Hirshel telling me he'd rather die at home with his family than die alone in a hospital room. "The problem is deciding when to stop fighting," my friend explained. "Sometimes people write themselves off too soon and give in too quickly. But if it looks as if nothing can be done for me, I hope they won't use heroic measures.

"There's a point where you have to distinguish between living and just existing," Hirshel continued. "But I could slip into a coma and not be able to make that decision. You may not be able to decide when the time comes. I just hope either Judi or I will be in control of the situation by then. Judi knows if it looks hopeless and if I'm in pain I should be allowed to have the dignity of a decent death."

The once-clear boundary between life and death is blurred. We used to define death as the cessation of breathing and heartbeat. But today we can mechanically sustain a patient's heart even though all brain waves have stopped. Is this a real "life," or is it mere "medical maintainance"? Now we can keep comatose patients "alive" for years, even though they can't speak, reason, perform normal bodily functions, or respond to outside stimuli. Is such a "life" still a gift from God?

Once we complained life was too brief. Now people argue life is sometimes too long, unnecessarily extended without the possibility of a cure, and devoid of all that makes living worthwhile. Once we unconditionally welcomed medical technology for its promises of cure and comfort, but for many today it has become an enemy that artificially sustains a life stripped of all quality.

April 6, 1984

Where is my remission? I guess it's coming to an end. Only a temporary stay.

Why did this have to happen now, one week before Rachel's Bat Mitzvah? We've been looking forward to it so much. Couldn't this damned leukemia have waited just a little while longer? Why does fate—or is it God—have to be so cruel? What a blow!

My children used to play the board game "Chutes and Ladders" when they were younger. One minute you're at the finish line nearly winning and the next second you're sliding back on a big chute to the beginning of the board and you've lost. I've decided that life is just like that. One minute you're up at the top and the next minute you're sliding down to the bottom.

Today while Judi was driving us back to Newburgh from our appointment with the specialist in Albany, she started to cry. Her mascara was running all over. The tears were just gushing out. I was afraid we'd have an automobile accident. I reached over and put my arm around her to comfort her. I guess reality hit her. It was like a backlash of all she has gone through. We were both sharing the same feeling—is this it?

Judi has never cried like that before, at least not in front of me. Her eyes mist over when someone does something nice for us and she realizes they really care. But she's never totally broken down before. That tough exterior is cracking. She said to me "Hirshel, I'm crying because I feel bad because you can't do anything about it. I feel helpless."

"I can do something, Judi," I told her. "I can fight it with this drug treatment."

Then it hit me again how devastating all this has been for Judi. She is under enormous pressure. I think it's harder for her than for me because she's just a spectator and she feels helpless. Everyone has said they could never endure what she has.

Our love has grown since my illness hit us. In this stark situation, stripped of our usual defenses, Judi and I have seen even more deeply into each other. Our marriage has really been put to a test, and our relationship has held fast and been strengthened. The marriage vows say, "in good fortune and in adversity." Well, we sure have hit the adversity part of the bargain, and Judi has really lived up to her vows.

Sometimes we think that famous Biblical proverb, "A woman of valor, who can find?" is trite. But this illness has shown me it's not. How many wives could cope with this? Most people would run away if they could. I know often marriages break up in situations like ours because couples can't deal with

134

the tensions and guilts and uncertainties that surface in a crisis like this.

A couple really has to be strongly committed to each other to pull through something like this together. Thank God I have somebody to share this with. The Song of Songs says, "Set me as a seal upon thy heart, for love is stronger than death."

Judaism holds marriage in such high regard that it compares the love between God and His people, Israel, to the relationship between husband and wife. The Jewish tradition insists that marriage is the best way to fulfill the human sexual drive and need for love. In a passage in the Babylonian Talmud a sage counsels, "A man who does not have a wife lives without joy, without blessing, and without goodness." A later scholar added, "And without peace."

Of course the rabbis, always realists, recognized that marriage and family life are full of complexities and pitfalls. They offer lots of advice—some of it very humorous—about how to settle conflicts between husband and wife, spouses and in-laws, and parents and children.

I couldn't cope with all this tumult in my life without Judi's endurance and love. Judi has held our family together during this crisis—all the while working at a full-time job! She has kept the girls going, trying to make their lives as normal as possible and still deal with their feelings too, and that hasn't been easy.

I can really see the rabbis were right when they said the wife sets the tone for the whole household, that "All depends on the woman." According to the Wisdom of Ben Sira, "A good wife makes a happy husband; she doubles the length of his life. A staunch wife is her husband's joy; he will live out his days in peace."

I know this puts a big burden on the wife, especially today, when most women work outside the home. Judi has always pursued her career since we've been married, and like other women she has trouble juggling her tasks and priorities. But she's committed to working because she is independent. She's always had her own life and identity outside of our relationship. The rabbis insisted that a good marriage must be based not only on love between a husband and wife but on mutual respect for each other, and I think this respect is enhanced when each spouse remains a whole person.

April 12, 1984

The septic tank gave out today. The sewage is backed up in our basement and our garage. Two days before Rachel's Bat Mitzvah! Is this unbelievable!? Everyone is coming in for the Bat Mitzvah tomorrow, and the house is a mess.

We'll have to recarpet the basement at least. And install a new septic tank in the backyard. That's going to cost a fortune. Right now, on top of all the Bat Mitzvah expenses. And we sure didn't need this aggravation now. There's enough on our minds with the last-minute Bat Mitzvah arrangements. This really is the last straw!

I know I shouldn't be so upset. I thought since my illness I had learned to put little things like this in the right perspective! Money isn't important, especially in light of my latest jolting medical setback. The only thing that really matters is that I lick this disease. Things like the septic tank will take care of themselves.

The cantor of Hirshel's congregation wants me there at least an hour early so we can go over the Bat Mitzvah service together. It takes about an hour and a half to drive from New York City to Newburgh, on the banks of the Hudson River. It's drizzling, so Marcia and I leave

Manhattan about 8 A.M. As we head north out into the country, the drizzle turns into rain and fog.

When we get to the synagogue, Hirshel, wearing blue jeans and unshaven, is moving tables into the social hall where the luncheon following the service and reception will be held. Judi is also dressed casually. She's setting up vases with flowers in them on each table. Rachel and Nina, also in blue jeans, are on top of a big ladder, putting up decorations. A custodian is sweeping the debris-covered floor. With the service scheduled to begin in an hour, my wife, always overorganized to a fault, is appalled at the chaos.

"Marcia, come home with us while we get dressed," Judi suggests. "There's nothing for you to do here, and I want to show you the big hole in our backyard. They came today to put in the new septic tank."

"Today?!"

"Yes, why not?" Judi laughs. "They're digging a huge hole with a big backhoe. The ground is total mud because of all the rain we've had. Men are tramping around my yard in work boots up to their hips. They turned our water off so Hirshel can't shave and we can't put on our makeup. Other than that," Judi says sarcastically, "everything is fine."

While Marcia goes with the Jaffes to their home about five minutes away from the synagogue, I hole up with the cantor in Hirshel's office to go over the procedure for the Bat Mitzvah.

Miraculously, everything and everyone is ready for the service. Judi is dressed in a lovely purple, pleated, flowing dress. Hirshel, very pale, wears a beige suit that unfortunately accentuates his chalky complexion. He had convinced the crew installing the new septic tank to turn on the water for a few minutes so he could shave. Rachel wears a pastel striped dress and little makeup.

She looks pristine and lovely. Nina, giggly and nervous, is adorable in a lacy white dress.

A Bar Mitzvah, for a boy, and Bat Mitzvah, sometimes called Bas Mitzvah, for a girl, is an occasion for family and friends of a thirteen-year-old to gather to share in the joy of watching this ritual transition from childhood into adulthood. As the child is called to the pulpit to chant a carefully prepared portion of the Torah reading designated for that particular Sabbath, the community acknowledges that this young person is now ready to enter into the responsibilities of adulthood in the Jewish community. Completing this *rite de passage* means he or she —in the Reform and Conservative branches of the religion—can now be regarded as a full member of the congregation and can be counted in the quorum of ten adults required to hold a public service.

While the Bar Mitzvah ceremony as we know it originated in the fourteenth century, the Bat Mitzvah ceremony for girls was started by Rabbi Mordecai Kaplan in the United States in this century. He wanted his five daughters to be able to share in the happy coming-of-age ceremony.

It is the most important day in a Jewish young person's religious life, and for the parent it is a day of pride mixed with sadness because childhood officially ends. On this day every parent wonders with some regret, as we did at our daughter's Bat Mitzvah last September, "Where has my little child gone? How did the years pass so quickly?"

This milestone in a child's life is generally a very happy day, but it can also be stressful because the entire family comes together. I read somewhere that the greatest number of illnesses, heart attacks, and strokes occur at family gatherings like this. I am thinking this morning that while this is an especially joyful time for Hirshel's family because he has survived his illness to celebrate it with them, it must also be difficult because of his uncertain prognosis.

Jews break a glass at the conclusion of every wedding ceremony to recall the destruction of the second Temple by the Romans in the year 70 C.E., an event that caused great sorrow to our people. This custom is a reminder that happy occasions in life are usually mixed with sadness, that life is always a bittersweet combination of both. Rachel's Bat Mitzvah today is certainly an example, for Hirshel's ever-present illness casts a dark shadow over the otherwise sunny day and adds a special poignancy to it.

April 14, 1984

Well, it's all over—the ceremony, the reception, the luncheon. Nearly everybody has gone home. After so much planning it's hard to believe it went by so quickly.

After such a horrible start everything turned out beautifully. It's amazing—it all worked out!

At first it seemed like everything was conspiring to go wrong: the septic tank, this gigantic gaping hole in the backyard. I could easily have said, "That's my life, one gaping hole." I started to shave and suddenly the guy is yelling, "No water, don't use the water." I thought, "Here I am trying to get ready for one of the biggest days in my life and I can't even shave!"

Then when we got over to the synagogue, I discovered the tables weren't in the social hall for the luncheon as they were supposed to be. I had to get them from the religious school, where the custodian had set them up for the kids' model seder tomorrow morning. It's right before Passover, and the temple isn't functioning. The custodian is half asleep in the youth lounge, where he is secretly harboring a three-legged cat, and

I have to fight to get tables for my own daughter's Bat Mitzvah luncheon. I had to set up the tables and chairs myself.

About half an hour before the service was supposed to start my parents telephoned the temple from a nearby gas station to say their car stalled in the middle of an intersection. My neighbor went to pick them up and found my dad almost not wanting to leave the gas station because he's worrying about what's going to happen to his car. Then we got another telephone call at the temple, from Judi's brother, Steve. He was at a mall trying to buy a new pair of slacks because his girl friend decided the pair he brought along didn't fit quite right.

But the moment the service started everything somehow fell into place. All the tensions disappeared and everybody was relaxed. I could relax too because Jim was officiating, so I could sit with the congregation and really be just myself, a person, a Jew, a proud daddy.

As I sat in the sanctuary listening to the service, I realized what a wonderful congregational rabbi Jim is. I've never seen him officiate before. I've gotten so used to thinking of him as that prominent American Jewish Committee personality who's in the newspapers and on TV and radio all the time that I forgot he really is a rabbi. Afterward everybody came up to me and said, "That rabbi is wonderful; who is he?" Jim really made the whole thing.

At the beginning of the service Jim talked about parents coping with adolescents. He said, "Fasten your seat belts, you're going through the turbulent teenage years." I thought, "Gee, he's really good." He has an informal manner that put everyone at ease.

And since Jim has been a friend of mine and my family for so long he brought a great warmth to the whole service. When he called members of my family to the pulpit individually to read their blessings over the Torah before and after Rachel read from it, he called them by their first names. He said, "Everybody is a Jaffe, we don't need to use last names." These weren't characters from a Hollywood cast; they were real people he knows or has heard about from me. It made the ceremony a personal experience for everybody there.

It flashed back to me as I listened to Jim this morning that in a strange way he was responsible for my meeting Judi. When I succeeded Jim as the assistant rabbi in Kansas City, he gave me his little black book with all the single girls' telephone numbers in it. It didn't have Judi's name in it. Jim knew her, but he thought she was too young to date.

But Judi's friend was in his little black book, and when Judi realized she wasn't in it she said to herself, "Hah, my friend is in the book and I'm not? That does it." So when she heard there was a new, young, single rabbi in town, she made it her business to come to services one Friday night to look me over. That's so like Judi, to take the first step! After services she came up to me and introduced herself. Her long hair was jet-black, and she looked at me with those big dark eyes you can drown in, and that was it for me. I thought she was alluring and fresh and rare. She is so beautiful. People have mistaken her at first glance for Elizabeth Taylor.

During the Bat Mitzvah service this morning I tried not to think about my leukemia. I didn't want anything to spoil this day for me. But how can you avoid dwelling on it? You can't program yourself. I'm living life and having very happy moments like this, but the balloon pops every once in a while and I worry what my next blood test will show.

I was wondering if Jim would mention my illness. He didn't. It wasn't necessary—I think it was uppermost in everybody's mind. He did say one thing, though, something like, "We all know the struggles the Jaffes have gone through to reach this day." Then Jim said something so beautiful. He said, "But after a troubled time you burst through to the blue skies."

His words "blue skies" evoked so many images for me. I remembered lying in the hospital after my spleenectomy and

*seeing little airplanes through my window and longing to be
free of my hospital prison. And I remembered dropping down
onto the beach on Martha's Vineyard in a beautiful multicol-
ored parachute pulled by a tow rope attached to a speeding
jeep. When they let go of the tow rope at two thousand feet,
I felt really free as I floated back to earth. So Jim used a very
meaningful and apt image.*

*When he said those things, Judi and I were up on the pulpit.
We could look out to about six rows in the congregation, and
I whispered, "Judi, the entire fifth row is breaking up." All the
women were crying. So were some of the men.*

*And, of course, all through the service the "Shehecheyanu"
kept running through my mind. For months I've been thinking, "I have to make it to Rachel's Bat Mitzvah." I didn't
think, "Let me live," but I said, "Dammit, I'm going to make
it, because I want to hear that line, say that line, feel that line:
'Thank you, God, for keeping me alive and sustaining me and
letting me reach this day.'"*

*This morning when the day had finally come it wasn't even
necessary to utter the prayer. Just being there was a "Shehecheyanu." I was there, and so was everybody else. I saw the
doctor who discovered my leukemia when he looked through
his microscope. And my surgeon friend who pushed me to get
a checkup when I told him I didn't feel well. I saw all my
friends who have been so wonderful. The whole cast of characters was there, but in a much different situation. It was staggering.*

*But, really, I didn't let my thoughts dwell on my illness this
morning. I was too elated.*

*I think the best part of the day was seeing how proud and
happy Judi was. Judi was more a mother and more real today
than I have ever seen her. She just beamed when Rachel,
looking so beautiful and radiant, recited her Torah portion
and gave her little speech. It was her child, her scene, and she
was totally caught up in it.*

*During the ceremony this morning I also remembered the
Rosh Hashana prayer that asks, "Who shall live and who shall
die?" I thought, "I shall live in spite of what happens." I'm
not saying I'm physically going to live. Who knows? But for
whatever time I have left I won't live as if I were haunted. No,
I'll live fully and completely.*

*My physical life is diminished, my bone marrow is overrun
with diseased cells, and my immune system is vulnerable. But
I feel spiritually I'm more of a person now, finally, that I am
in the blue skies. I'm holding up my family. I feel more in
command of things. I've yielded something to eternity, which
is my medical fate. You can't change that.*

But, strangely, somehow I feel more alive.

By facing death I am learning how to live.

11

〜〜〜

May 10, 1984

Today I begin taking the leukeran pills twice a day. Here's hoping. . . .

July 10, 1984

I had to give up my Greenhaven Prison chaplaincy. I just don't have the energy for it. I have to put all my strength into my Newburgh congregation now. I owe them that. The prisoners sent me cards and letters wishing me luck when they found out I was leaving. I was touched.

In August we're going to Martha's Vineyard for three weeks. Maybe a good vacation will help me get some of my strength back.

July 31, 1984

Two weeks ago we got some shocking news. One of the people killed in that shooting in the McDonald's restaurant near San Diego was a young woman I had just married to a congregant from Newburgh three weeks earlier! A bride of three weeks wiped out with twenty others in this senseless

145

slaughter! I remember how radiant and beautiful she was at her wedding. Now I am trying to help the stunned groom get through this devastating tragedy.

Everyone wants to know why this happened. They want to know what explanation Judaism can offer. They challenge me, they ask, "Well, Rabbi, what do you think?" They aren't being antagonistic or hostile; they genuinely want to know. My dazed congregants wonder how God could allow a crazed man like the one who opened fire at that McDonald's to massacre innocent people. Why does He bring this torment to their families and friends? Is there a reason, or is it all meaningless?

I feel so inadequate. What can I tell this distraught young man robbed of his future with the woman he loved so much? What can I tell others who bear terrible losses? What words can comfort them? And dammit, why should I even have to try? I'm only human—I want to run away from sorrow, I don't want constantly to face these tragedies. Why should I always have to try to answer these difficult questions?

It's at times like this that I wonder why I ever became a rabbi. Do I have the strength to cope with this? How can I be a rabbi when I can't even deal with my own doubts and confusions brought on by my illness? Maybe I should have been something else. Maybe Jim is right, I'd be better off in another profession now. But have I ever measured up to this superhuman task?

Yet, really, who does? And, in spite of my doubts I am a rabbi, and I know more than ever that I want to be one for the rest of my life. So I feel compelled to wrestle with these issues and try to give people answers, especially since now I'm agonizing too because of my leukemia.

I recite all the traditional philosophical and Jewish responses to the problem of evil I've thought about since rabbinical school. But they usually don't help people. Sometimes I say, "I have no other answers for you. I've been asking these same questions myself since my illness, and I can't come up with satisfying explanations for myself, so how can I help you?" One mourner told me, "Rabbi, it's partly because of your illness that I come to you for answers. I feel you have something to give me, more since your illness than before."

Maybe she's right. Maybe that is the reason for my illness —that now I do have something to give to people that I didn't have before. That now, even if I can't answer their agonized questions of "Why?", at least I can give them my real understanding and concern, at least I can give them myself.

August 6, 1984

The Vineyard is beautiful and relaxing as always. My spirits are good even though my energy is limited. Sometimes it's almost too much for me to walk the two hundred yards down to the beach. It tires me out to climb the stairs from the beach to our deck.

We are having a lot of company. In the afternoons I excuse myself from our guests and lie down to watch the spectacular Summer Olympics on television. Ironically, about a year ago Judi and I planned to buy tickets for the games and make the trip to Los Angeles to see them. I'm glad we didn't—I couldn't make that trip now.

It's difficult for me to watch these magnificent young athletes perform while I'm fighting now for enough energy just to limp through the day. I feel like warning these young people, telling them, "Enjoy it while you can . . . don't think your wonderful bodies will last forever."

Today a friend flew me in his private plane from the Vineyard to a Cape Cod hospital in Hyannis so I could get my blood tested. The counts haven't dropped much from three weeks ago, when they were monitored by my hematologist at home. But they haven't risen either. I still believe they'll pick up.

147

New blood tests show the leukeran is still not raising my counts. My hematologist is becoming more concerned. I'm getting even more anemic, and the doctors say the leukeran is causing that. They did tell me the leukeran might depress my blood counts and make me worse before it helps me.

My hematologist thinks we should stop the leukeran now, even though I'm supposed to take it for twelve more weeks. It's difficult to decide what to do because if I go off the leukeran the only treatment left is interferon. I really want to complete the six months of leukeran—I don't want to go off it before we give it a chance to work. But it seems to be hurting me. The doctors can't afford to let my counts slide down too far now. It's too dangerous for me.

I might need a blood transfusion because of my low red cell count. My white cell count is dropping below 1500, and normal is 5000. I don't have much immunity in my system so my body can't fight off routine illnesses. Any infection could finish me off, so I have to be careful about making physical contact with people. Here I am, a rabbi, and I can't even kiss people after services to wish them a "Good Shabbas," or embrace them. I have to worry about what I might catch.

I'm beginning to wonder how I'll ever get through the High Holiday services this year. Is this some plan by God? It seems like every High Holiday season I face a new medical crisis.

I just had another blood test, and my count is very disappointing. My hematologist is upset—we have developed a close relationship. We called the hairy-cell leukemia specialist in Chicago. He agrees the leukeran may not be working. He had predicted it would start to raise my counts by Rosh Hashana, but Rosh Hashana has come and gone. The leukeran hasn't raised my counts; it seems to be making me worse.

We three decided on the telephone to abandon the leukeran treatment. I will go out to Chicago in a month to begin interferon injections. We have to wait that long because they have to allow time for the leukeran to get cleaned out of my body before they can start putting interferon into it.

Judi and I are scheduled to go out to Chicago on October twenty-ninth. Hope I can hold out until then.

October 3, 1984

What a long day.

My doctor decided I had to have a blood transfusion or I wouldn't have the energy to get through Yom Kippur in a few days. I went in for the transfusion today. I thought it would be a breeze. But nothing is ever simple these days. I should know that by now.

It took seven hours for me to get two units of red blood cells. My veins are so delicate they had to keep slowing down the rate of the transfusion because it was so painful. And in the middle of everything the machine broke down and they had to send for another one. I didn't bring a book to read or a radio or anything, so I just lay there for seven hours counting spots in the ceiling. That's hard to do. But since I've been hit with this illness I've had to learn to have patience.

Now I'm starting to have fevers of almost 101 degrees. They come on me when I'm in bed, and I wake up with these awful night sweats. The doctors say it will be dangerous for me if the fevers get any higher.

I still have that irritating cough. The doctors think it might be caused by nerves.

～～～～

"I'm in the hospital again, Jim," Hirshel explains to me on the telephone. "My doctor's very worried about the fevers I've been having at night, and he wants to find out what's causing them. He's afraid I have an infection, which could wipe me out right now because my white count is so low and my immune system isn't giving me any protection. So they're running tests on me here and giving me antibiotics intravenously.

"The doctor wanted to put me in the hospital the day before Yom Kippur, but I told him I just couldn't miss Yom Kippur services. He finally relented when he realized how important it was for me to lead my congregation.

"I barely made it through the services. I had a fever all day. I don't know how I did it, sheer willpower, I guess. Somehow I found the strength to do it. I just knew that I had to, and so I pushed myself, forced myself to keep going. But it took everything out of me.

"I didn't fast, of course. Even my kids reminded me you don't have to fast if you're sick. At noon I went home and rested and ate lunch. Judi plied me with liquids all day to keep my fever down. She has been so concerned and is taking such good care of me. Judi's very upset by my fevers and low blood counts, and she's getting cynical about everything that's going wrong.

"But it's funny, Jim. Even though I had so little physical energy, I felt very strong spiritually. I don't know why—I guess because I feel my physical situation deteriorating so much—but during these High Holidays I gave the best and most honest sermons of my life. I talked about hope and survival in the face of adversity and reaching out to those who need us.

"I said to myself, 'This is it, Hirshel, you have to give your all.' All my masks are stripped away, and I can say everything I'm really thinking now. I guess it's because

I have nothing to lose. It sounds strange, but there's a real freedom in that. I'm not nervous anymore about how people will receive my sermons—will somebody get mad at me if I say something they don't like? I made some very strong statements about marital infidelity, and Judi told me some people in the congregation winced. But mainly they responded to my deep feelings and convictions. . . . I don't know when I'll get out of here. We might have to miss your big fiftieth birthday party, Jim. I'm sorry. We were looking forward to it."

I am struck by the irony of the situation: Marcia and I are planning a large birthday party to mark my mid-life milestone at the very time Hirshel is fighting for his life. I almost feel guilty about our celebration. Although we don't put it into words, both Hirshel and I know that he may not make it to his fiftieth birthday.

About a week later we drive upstate to visit Hirshel on a beautiful, unseasonably warm autumn day. The vivid oranges, yellows, and reds of the trees that line the highway are at their peak.

Hirshel is in a small room, alone. We are happy and a little surprised to see him looking so well. You'd never know he was ill, except that he's pale. He is lying down on the bed staring up at the ceiling, looking very relaxed and serene, with earphones in his ears.

"I'm listening to Zalman Schacter's healing tape," Hirshel explains. "He sent it to me along with his books. I told him about my illness in a long phone conversation a few weeks ago, and he gave me his long-distance blessing for health. You know, nineteen years ago this same rabbi gave me a wedding blessing right before I married Judi."

Rabbi Zalman Schacter is a modern-day mystic who believes in the power of personal, repetitive prayer to help heal the body. Hirshel plays us a sample of the tape.

We hear Rabbi Schacter repeat over and over in a gentle voice four Hebrew words, "*El na, rafah na,*" which mean, "O God, please heal us now." Then he says phrases like "Think of yourself by a quiet brook. . . . Let your soul be quieted so you can find inner peace. . . ." Schacter's deep, soothing voice does have a calming effect, and I can see that his charismatic personality might take powerful hold.

We "modern" Jews tend to forget that mystical traditions are a very important part of our religion. For many years "rational" Jews belittled and ridiculed Jewish mysticism as somewhat primitive, even embarrassing. But within the past thirty years this deep stream of Jewish thought was rediscovered by a "rational" modern Jew, the late Gershom Scholem. Because of his stunning scholarship and because we've learned a great deal about the inextricable connection between mind and body, the Jewish mystical tradition is now taken much more seriously. And thinkers like Zalman Schacter are helping to revive it.

"Hirshel, it's a little out of character for you to be indulging in this sort of thing," I joke. "And you know, the rabbis always said don't use faith healing or witchcraft to get well. We should use only the latest scientific medical techniques."

"That's true, Jim, but Rabbi Schacter would never want us to use these tapes instead of medicine. And I think now we realize the rabbis' distinction between scientific medical care and miracles is too strict. The more we advance medically the more we realize we can't draw such a neat line between miracles and science when it comes to the human body. There are just too many things about it we don't understand."

"I guess you're right. What we used to call witchcraft

today we can see as close interaction between the mind and body. What we used to call a miracle is often the power of faith or prayer. . . . So how are they treating you in this hospital?"

"I'm getting very good care here," Hirshel says. "The nurses are just wonderful. Of course there are the usual funny incidents. The first night I was here an alcoholic with the DT's was screaming all night. Then once in the middle of the night there was a big crash. Somebody's bed had collapsed. I'm lonely, though. I don't even have a roommate. I have to be in isolation so I won't pick up any germs. I have to wear a mask when I walk around the halls. The doctors joked and said hospitals are the best places in the world to pick up germs."

"Are you still having the fevers?" Marcia asks.

"Yes. They debilitate me. They come on me at night and I can't sleep too well. They haven't found out what's causing them yet. They're giving me every test they can. We have to get rid of the fevers because I can't get the interferon until they're gone. So there's a crucial time element here. I've stopped taking the leukeran, so my only chance to fight the disease now is the interferon. I just have to make it to Chicago by November first to start the interferon treatments."

Hirshel is in the upstate New York hospital for a total of sixteen days. My friend is hit with an array of strong antibiotic drugs to combat the fevers, and has numerous blood workups to try to find out what is causing them. But nothing shows up on the tests, and things are getting worse.

Suddenly Hirshel's hematologist decides to send him out to the hospital in Chicago where he is scheduled to begin the interferon injections. Perhaps, he reasons, the specialist in hairy-cell leukemia with whom he has been

153

consulting, the man under whose guidance the experimental drug interferon will be administered, can locate the source of Hirshel's mysterious fevers.

October 26, 1984

I am writing this on the airplane, waiting to take off for Chicago.

The doctors moved up the date for Judi and me to go to Chicago. I didn't even go home. Judi packed a suitcase for me, and an ambulance took us directly from the hospital to Stewart Airport, near Newburgh, for our special flight.

Judi and I are the only passengers on this private jet. It's an "Angel of Mercy" flight a compassionate businessman provides free for cancer patients who must travel to receive medical attention. It's wonderful to know that somebody cares. We need that morale boost right now, because on top of everything else Judi lost her purse with all her money and credit cards last night. Just what we needed right now!

This is so ironic. When the American hostages were freed from Teheran, they flew to Stewart Airport, and I was here to greet them when they landed in January 1981. Now, almost four years later, I am leaving from the same airport to try to save my own life.

During the summer I was invited to speak at a Polish-American–American Jewish Committee conference in Chicago on October twenty-sixth. I thought then this one-day trip to Chicago would be just another in-and-out journey that is so much a part of my professional duties. How could I know that this would be the very day Hirshel and Judi arrived in Chicago to check into the hospital? And an even bigger coincidence: I'm scheduled to return to Chicago for another conference on November first, the day Hirshel's supposed to start his interferon regimen. Our lives have always intersected, and now we'll be together on these two crucial days in Hirshel's life. Maybe I'm fated to watch over my friend!

My speech to the Polish-Jewish conference ends about 3 P.M. As I hurry over to Hirshel's hospital a few blocks away, college students rush past me, many with Mondale/Ferraro buttons on their coats. Young men and women hold hands walking together across the newly fallen autumn leaves. As one couple passes me, I catch a piece of their conversation about plans for the upcoming weekend. I think, "So many private passions are being played out before me: students in love and a rabbi battling for his life . . . all in the same block."

Hirshel's building is a large, modern, green-and-white glass-box tower that looks like something from a science fiction movie. The sun reflects off it in the late October afternoon. It is sterile and icy cold in style, and it seems out of character with the older, somehow friendlier buildings that surround it.

I rush by the receptionist mumbling something about being a rabbi, which always gives me access to hospitals any time of the day or night. I take a carpeted elevator to the sixth floor, the top of the hospital, and move quickly toward Hirshel's room. As I go through the corridor, my eyes wander and I glance into each room, an old habit I acquired when I was a congregational rabbi. I like to get the feel of the ward or floor I'm visiting.

Even though I am a seasoned hospital visitor, today I am very depressed. This hospital is different, clearly a cancer ward. The few visitors I encounter seem dazed and melancholy. The faces of the patients are ashen and taut, their cheeks are pinched and their eyes mournful.

Finally I reach the corner room and quickly look in, expecting to find Hirshel and Judi. But instead two men are cleaning the room, changing the sheets, and spraying disinfectant everywhere.

"Where's the patient, Rabbi Jaffe?" I ask them.

"Don't know. We just clean."

I am afraid to ask them what happened to the patient who was in the bed before. Someone at the nurse's station, which looks like a cross between a sleek bank lobby and an airline ticket counter, informs me that Rabbi Jaffe is in the lobby waiting to be admitted.

As I walk back to the elevators to go down to the waiting room, I stop for a moment and peer into an open conference room. A man in a white medical jacket is addressing a group of eight or ten people paying very close attention to him. One of the physicians glares at me and I hurry on.

The waiting room fits in perfectly with the sterilized motif of the building. Padded benches face each other at right angles, and artificial palms provide screens of semi-privacy. Judi is sitting alone on one of the benches reading a newspaper.

"Hi, Jim. Hirshel is looking around the gift shop," Judi says. "We're really upset. We've heard that the specialist we came out to see is still in San Francisco today and won't be back until tomorrow. Another day lost for Hirshel."

"What does the specialist look like?" I ask her.

She's never met him, but she relates the description Hirshel has given her.

"Judi, I saw either him or his double a few minutes ago in a conference room on Hirshel's floor."

Just then the physician I had seen approaches us, trailed by a very pregnant associate. He explains he has just arrived from California and has already had a staff meeting to discuss Hirshel's case. "Where's the rabbi?" he asks.

"He's in the gift shop. I'm Judi Jaffe."

Like two bloodhounds, the physicians run into the shop and retrieve Hirshel. Much paler than the last time I saw him, in the other hospital, Hirshel embraces me weakly, and the five of us go back up to the sixth floor.

After Hirshel is settled in his room, I leave the Jaffes alone with the doctors so they can discuss their next course of action. As I step into the fresh autumn air and hail a taxi to take me to the airport and home, I am relieved to be out of the depressing cancer ward and thankful I can walk out of the hospital freely. How much we take for granted when we are healthy!

But I am almost ashamed of my selfish feelings of relief, for I am leaving my good friend behind to face his uncertain fate.

12

~~~~~~~

During the flight from Chicago to New York I scan an article Hirshel gave me about hairy-cell leukemia his doctor and a colleague wrote. Surprisingly, I understand the monograph quite well. The bottom line, according to Hirshel's specialist, one of the world's leading experts on his disease, is that no one knows very much about it.

They do know the illness strikes men much more frequently than women, and most victims are in their forties, Hirshel's age. The patient's lifespan is uncertain. Because the body's immune system is badly weakened by the disease, infection is the leading cause of death for hairy-cell leukemia patients. I realize now they must discover what's causing Hirshel's high fevers.

Suddenly I am exhausted from my long conference and the emotional strain of visiting my friend. I lean my head back on the headrest and close my eyes. Images of those pale patients—young and old—with their haunting eyes float into my mind. Will Hirshel soon be one of them? Will he look like that? Will he have to suffer with excruciating pain? How will interferon affect him? Will Hirshel give up the treatments if the drug causes him too much agony? Will he ever decide to let his disease just take its course and allow himself some final peace and dignity? Will Judi or others have to make these decisions for him?

More families are facing heartbreaking situations concerning care of their loved ones. Every day we read stories about doctors, nurses, or family members "pulling the plug" on terminally ill or brain-dead patients. The term "negotiated death" is now part of our vocabulary. We are often torn between the religious commitment to prolong life and our personal anguish when we see pain. Hirshel and I, like all other clergy, have seen some families literally torn apart when they face these wrenching questions, and now I fear Hirshel himself could soon be wrestling with them.

The medical and legal communities and even the government are gearing up to deal with these complex moral and social questions raised by the new and rapidly growing medical technology. Coincidentally, I have just been appointed by Governor Mario Cuomo to a Task Force on Life and the Law set up to study these issues and to recommend appropriate legislation for the state of New York. Debates are taking place that try to reconcile traditional religion's views about the sanctity of life with modern technology's new options. Will the Jewish tradition, I wonder, be able to offer guidance to Hirshel and his family on these complex and agonizing issues?

Religious thinkers today must choose between two basic positions. The argument hinges on an acceptable definition of life and when it stops being meaningful. One position holds that since we are created in God's image, all human life is sacred, so extending a person's life for even a few seconds is as valid and worthwhile as extending it for decades.

The other view maintains that each medical case should be reviewed individually, that the quality of life can be defined and evaluated by a set of verifiable stan-

160

dards, such as: Is the patient conscious? Can he feel and reason? According to these criteria, for example, a "brain-dead" person who has no consciousness no longer has a meaningful life, and therefore one is not religiously obligated to try to sustain it.

Rabbi Maurice Lamm calls these alternative positions the "sanctity of life" argument and the "quality of life" argument.

Because Judaism teaches that every human life is infinitely valuable and we must make every effort to save it, the tradition emphasizes the "sanctity of life" argument, or the first position. According to Jewish law, if we don't do everything possible to save or prolong life, we are shortening or terminating it, which is forbidden.

Because of the complexities of modern medical technology, however, today some Jews now advocate the other position, the "quality of life" argument. While they admit the "sanctity of life" view is ethically admirable, they assert it does not apply to every situation, arguing that God does not require us to extend a meaningless life of pain without realistic expectation of recovery.

But if you don't act to prolong life, aren't you really shortening it? The Jewish religion is staunchly opposed to doing anything that even slightly hastens death. Life is a gift from God, who alone determines how and when death will come. Rabbi Joseph Caro declared, "We are not permitted to close the eyes of a person who is near death, lest one cut off even a fraction of life." You are not allowed to remove a pillow or a cushion from a dying person if such an act will in any way speed up death. You cannot withhold food and necessary medicine from a patient.

Roman Catholic thinkers have tried to solve these problems by distinguishing between "heroic" and "ordinary" medical procedures. They generally oppose un-

161

dertaking "heroic" procedures, while advocating "ordinary" procedures. But organ transplants, brain tumor operations, and use of kidney machines, once considered "heroic" measures, are today "ordinary." The once clear difference between "heroic" and "ordinary" measures has faded and no longer offers a guideline.

Although Jewish scholars do not use the terms "heroic" and "ordinary" medical procedures, they wrestle with the same problems. Dr. Fred Rosner, a professor at Yeshiva University's Albert Einstein School of Medicine, cites a typical cancer case to illustrate this dilemma. A nine-year-old girl has leukemia, and her only hope— a long shot—is a bone marrow transplant with the girl's father as the donor. Should surgeons perform such a hazardous operation? Should the girl's age be a factor in reaching a decision? Does Judaism permit the "risk/benefit" factor to enter into the discussion? May there be/must there be a transplant operation according to Jewish law? Who must give consent to such a risky procedure?

Rosner cites Rabbi Moshe Feinstein, one of the leading Orthodox Jewish authorities in the world, who says, "Do the dangerous surgery; perhaps it will succeed. It is a risk worth taking." Any act that will prolong life is permitted. The Talmudic rabbis say if a patient has exhausted all conventional medical treatment—you must try standard treatment first—you may take a chance by performing risky surgery or using extraordinary measures, even if the experimental treatment might shorten the person's life in the long run.

According to author Francine Klagsbrun, such discussions in the Talmud focused around the issue of whether or not "heathen" physicians—non-Jewish doctors who, the rabbis felt, employed idolatrous forms of magic in

162

their cures—may treat a Jew. The scholars concluded that if a critically ill patient will die without such treatment, it is permitted. Advises one Talmudic commentator, "When we are in doubt about whether a patient will live or die, we must not allow idolators to heal. But if the patient *certainly* will die, we may allow them to heal." So, in the face of certain and imminent death, one can permit even faith-healing techniques, a remarkable teaching since the Jewish tradition generally disapproves of all such forms of "nonscientific" medical treatments.

But if Judaism commands us to prolong life, does it also command us to prolong the process of dying? While we cannot hasten death in any way, must we force a terminally ill patient to live longer? When a medical cure is no longer possible, shouldn't we stop medical treatment and just try to make the patient's last days as comfortable as possible, placing him or her in a comfortable hospice, for example?

Rabbi Solomon Freehof, a leading Talmudic scholar, argues that while the Jewish tradition permits us to take risks to save a life, it doesn't allow us to prolong the process of dying. If the purpose of the risky operation is "to gain an hour or two of life, then it should not be performed." Physicians should operate only if there is a reasonable chance the patient's condition will significantly improve. Freehof rightly calls this area "murky and ambiguous," and, admitting the contradition of his position, says, "We must fight for every second of life actively, but we can be passive in the case of a terminally ill person."

Freehof and Rosner highlight the tension in Jewish thought between preserving life and not interfering with the natural process of dying. Judaism absolutely forbids killing by active intent and active euthanasia. But what about passive forms of euthanasia, such as removing a life-support system, refusing to resuscitate, or refusing to begin new medical or drug therapy on a patient? Is this morally and legally murder?

Suppose no bone marrow transplant is performed on Rosner's hypothetical nine-year-old leukemia victim and she soon dies. Is this hastening death, killing by neglect? Or is it simply not interfering with the process of dying? Are we commanded to prolong the process of dying when no cure is available?

The issue becomes even more complex when we talk about the removal of a life-support system from a patient who is terminally ill or in a coma. Here Judaism offers us some insights and guidelines.

Two dramatic Talmudic stories provide justification to remove such systems from the terminally ill. Because he taught the Torah, Roman authorities executed Rabbi Hananiah ben Teradyon, like many of his colleagues, by burning him alive at the stake. To prolong the rabbi's torture, the Romans covered him with water-filled sponges to insure that death would not come quickly. As the fire grew hotter, Hananiah's students begged him to draw the fire into his throat, and by so doing take his own life and end his suffering. The rabbi refused to allow the fire to enter his throat to hasten his own death. But he did permit a Roman soldier to remove the sponges from him, and soon afterward the rabbi died.

It is a subtle but critical point. The dying rabbi would not allow the fire to enter his throat—an active step—but he did permit the removal of the sponges, his primitive life-support system—a passive act. The soldier allowed the rabbi, obviously in a "terminal" situation, to die naturally and without an outside "life-support system."

The Talmudic scholars of course commend the rabbi for his brave martyrdom, but surprisingly also praise the unknown Roman soldier for removing the sponges, and accord both the rabbi and the soldier an honored place in the world to come. The story teaches that you are rewarded for easing the pain of a dying person. Those with no hope of escaping death can request that the dying process be shortened, although they cannot take steps themselves to shorten their lives.

In the second story the great Talmudic authority Rabbi Yehudah Ha Nasi, Judah the Prince, lay dying in his house, while his adoring students gathered outside to pray for his recovery. Since, according to the Jewish tradition, prayers for the sick are just as effective as medical treatment, the students' petitions to God provided a kind of life-support system for the patient.

Judah's agony worsened. His female attendant, acutely aware of her master's intense suffering, in desperation took a large earthen jar to the roof of the rabbi's house and hurled it to the ground below, where it shattered into many pieces. Stunned by the noise, the students momentarily stopped their prayers, thereby withdrawing the emotional "support system." The Talmud recounts that in that period of silence, Judah Ha Nasi died. It praises the attendant, even though her behavior hastened Judah's death.

In the much earlier Biblical account of King Saul, the Israelite leader is gravely wounded in battle and, fearing he will fall into his enemies' hands alive, asks an Amalekite to kill him with a sword. The soldier carries out Saul's request and ends his agony. Biblical commentators writing many centuries later surprisingly do not condemn either Saul or his slayer, implying that easing a person's pain is a meritorious act.

According to Moses Isserles, a sixteenth-century scholar, one may remove obstacles to death, such as the chopping of wood outside a patient's home if the sound of the chopping acts as a stimulus. Isserles also permitted salt to be removed from a patient's tongue if it serves as a stimulus. Two centuries later another Jewish teacher warned, "Do not pray too hard that a soul will return, that is, revive from a coma, for the ill person can at best live only a few days, and during that time he will endure great pain."

However, we are confused because Isserles also taught the opposite: "If a person is near death, do not even remove the cushion or pillow under his head, lest it speed up death." And Moses Maimonides opposed all "passive euthanasia" actions: "He who kills a healthy person," the great scholar counseled, "and he who kills a sick person who is dying anyway, even if he is almost dead, all are guilty of murder!"

A thirteenth-century rabbi, Nissim Gerondi, taught that there can be no *active* hastening of death, but one can offer *prayers* to God for death. Most Jewish authorities do permit a terminal patient to pray for his own death, and also permit another to pray for it, since such a request requires God, not a human being, to end the life. There is a difference between praying to hasten death and actually acting to bring it about.

Despite these confusing questions and answers, modern Jewish scholarship does provide some guideliness for these difficult bio-ethical problems. One can withhold medical treatment from the terminally ill if it is very painful and stressful and will prolong dying rather than living. However, in such cases it should be the patient's decision and not the family's or the doctor's, if the patient is willing and able to decide. A patient may refuse resuscitation and refuse to initiate all further treatment, but cannot refuse to eat. One should give all painkilling drugs, including morphine and other narcotics, if they will make the patient more comfortable. When patients cannot be cured, it is our duty, according to the Jewish tradition, to try to comfort them and ease their pain. Says Dr. Rosner, "When physicians recognize they have no more to offer medically, they no longer have the license to treat.... There is a point where we just must learn to ease pain better." "Heroic" methods can be offered to the patient if they do not cause pain or risk death.

October 31, 1984

Early this morning when the doctors made their rounds, I said to them, "My God, I think these antibiotics are doing something to me! Something is happening to my body!" They burst into laughter. I was wearing the Frankenstein-monster mask Judi bought me for Halloween. It is so real-looking. I kept it on all day as the other nurses and the physicians came into my room, and they all got hysterical. This is such a grim floor I think the staff is thankful for any excuse to laugh.

With all my years of visiting patients as a rabbi, I've never seen anything like this place. I know I'm a patient, I'm part of it, but I can still stand outside of myself and look at this ward like an outsider.

Almost everyone on this floor has cancer. There's a quietness here. There are empty cans of chemicals from the chemotherapy treatments lying in trash bins in the corridors. Patients wander slowly up and down the halls, many completely bald and wearing surgical masks. I'm afraid to look in the rooms when I walk around, because I know I'll see people who are much worse off than I am.

One scene is especially wrenching. A sixteen-year-old boy is dying of lymphoma. His parents are here all day long every day, continually walking him up and down the halls. Each parent holds onto one of the boy's arms while he leans on them. It is so sad I can hardly bear to look at them.

The doctors are giving me antibiotics intravenously and performing every test they know to find what's causing my fevers. They are sticking so many needles into me I feel like the proverbial pincushion. The fevers still come mostly at night and disappear during the day. But they are quite high, and I have restless and sleepless nights. Sometimes they have to change my sheets five times during the night.

I'm trying to be patient and keep up my spirits. Last Sunday was the New York City Marathon, and I watched the runners on my little TV set. It seems like a million years since I ran in it. Has it really been only six years? What good is it to wish I were my old self again, that I could push my body to make that run?

Then there's the boredom to cope with. I'm in a single room as I was in the other hospital so I won't catch anything. Thank God Judi is here to talk to most of the day. She arranged to take time off from her job, and we left the kids with my folks for a few days.

I really need her here with me.

November 1, 1984

Today is the day I was scheduled to begin the interferon. They can't give it to me because of the fevers. I'm so disappointed. They don't know when we can start. Still no clue as to what's causing the fevers. They keep giving me different antibiotics, hoping one of them will counteract the infection.

Jim came to visit me again today. I talk to Marcia in New

York every day by telephone, but it's not the same as having somebody here. God, I realize again how important it is to have an emotional support system. It's almost as important as the medical staff.

Judi is much different here than she was when I was in the hospital for my spleenectomy two years ago. She's not covering up her feelings with her wry humor. She's here with me every day for hours, and she's very engrossed and involved with me. We have a beautiful relationship here, a strong bond. We can even cry together.

But I think she's getting restless. Yesterday she went to the Museum of Science and Industry for a few hours, and a couple of nights ago she went out to dinner with some old friends. She wants to be here in Chicago with me, but I know she's anxious to get back home too so she can get back to work and be with Rachel and Nina. Judi thought she'd be helping me get through my interferon treatments, but there's really nothing for her to do because we're just waiting for the results from my tests.

It's obvious now to my congregants that I won't be able to go back to work for a long time. So far they're managing to keep the synagogue running without me, and they are careful to let me know they aren't going to replace me.

Lay people are reading the services every week. Anyone can lead services; rabbis aren't really necessary. But I guess they do think of me as having a priestly function. My president said they had a long discussion about whether any of them should raise their arms and give the blessing to the congregation at the end of the service. They worried about whether anybody except the rabbi should do this. They finally decided the cantor could do it, so now he's giving the closing benediction.

It's funny—they're almost superstitious about these things. One woman told me, "Don't worry, Rabbi, nobody ever sits in your seat on the pulpit."

Frequently I hear those terrible beeping noises that mean "Staff come quick, there's an emergency." That indicates someone's life is in danger.

Somebody on the floor died last night. My door was open this morning and I saw them wheeling the body past my room.

I'm not going to look out into the hallway anymore.

November 6, 1984

Election Day. It's hard to believe that life still goes on out there while I'm at a standstill here just waiting.

Judi finally went home yesterday. We couldn't justify her staying here anymore. And the girls need her. God, I really miss my daughters. I think about them all the time and talk to them on the phone every night. They tell me all about their ski trips and school dances.

I'll have to get home without Judi by myself after they give me the interferon. If they ever give me the interferon. First they have to find out what's causing these fevers. Yesterday they took a liver biopsy. It was very painful—they inserted a needle into my side. But I had to go through it because they're testing me for a rare form of tuberculosis that has killed four hairy-cell leukemia patients.

My specialist said if they don't find a way to stop my dangerous fevers soon, they will apply to the drug company that makes interferon and to the FDA for "Compassionate Usage" of the drug. This would allow them to give it to me even though I have a fever. I love those words "Compassionate Usage." It's amazing how you can mask life-and-death matters with bureaucratic language!

The physicians and nurses here have been wonderful. They answer all my questions and always let me in on what's hap-

pening. Sometimes they tell me too much. When the specialist assured me, "Rabbi, we always find the cause of the fevers," I said to him, "Always?" He said, "Well, sometimes we don't find it until after the autopsy."

That really cheered me up! But it was I who kept pushing him for an answer, and, really, I do appreciate their honesty. The whole staff obviously cares about me. Maybe that's because I assert myself and they see me as a real individual. Like when I clowned around with that great Halloween mask.

The other night one of the young doctors came into my room and sat down in the chair near my bed and just talked to me for about an hour and a half. He put his head in his hands and said, "Rabbi, I wish to God I had found the answer to your disease." After he left I shed a few tears because he cared about me so much.

And my specialist, who's the head of this whole unit, telephones me from his home to talk to me if he's not at the hospital. The nurses said that is very unusual. Today when I told him I'm lonely because Judi went back to Newburgh, he got on the telephone and called up a rabbi friend he knows from summer camp years ago and practically ordered him to come over here and visit me.

Maybe being a rabbi singles me out and makes the staff notice me. Somehow word got out quickly that I was a clergyman, and it seems everybody here comes to me with their problems. Guess I can just never escape the counseling role. One of the nurses sat here the other day and told me all her family troubles. Other patients wander into my room to talk. Last night a man from down the hall, a Lutheran, asked me to pray for him. Now that people sense I have gone through so much with this disease, they seek me out more than ever.

The hospital staff even asked me to address a group of medical students on the emotional aspects of my disease. They want to know the real story of the patient as a person. The students seemed really enthralled by what I had to say. I felt

171

so fulfilled by the chance to influence these young potential healers, and happy I could repay this staff for my wonderful care.

For some reason I am able to touch people. Maybe everyone senses how calm and at peace I am. I know that I feel spiritually stronger than I ever have, and certainly far better able to cope psychologically with the ups and downs of my physical condition and with the vicissitudes of hospital life than I was when I first got sick two years ago.

November 7, 1984

I feel so alone here without Judi. We talk on the phone at all hours, and my parents call a lot too. I wish they could fly out from New York. I'm glad more friends have come to visit me here. Three local rabbis came today.

I scared them because I had a horrible case of chills while they were here. My entire body was shaking as if I had malaria. The doctors were giving me an antifungal drug to try to get rid of my fevers, but it wracked my body so much with these chills they decided it wasn't worth it, and they stopped it.

I don't like all these strong poisons going into my system. Who knows what they do to your body? But one of these days they might hit on the antibiotic that will help me. I'm locked in combat with this disease now, so I have to fight it with everything I can.

November 8, 1984

The "Compassionate Usage" permission came through. This morning I got my first shot of interferon.

I expected some horrible side effects immediately, but so far today I've felt nothing. Maybe for a change I'll be lucky. I just feel optimistic and elated that finally we're doing something that might help me.

I am praying now that this strange new drug will work its magic.

13

~~~~~

"I'm home, Jim."

"What a surprise! That's great."

'They let me go home after I learned how to give myself the interferon shots. Now Judi gives them to me. I get three shots a week. The doctors are hopeful this new drug will stem the disease. But there really aren't many statistics. So few patients have used it that numbers don't mean much. The program just began in 1983, and only about sixty people are using interferon throughout the country, thirty of us in this Chicago program. I'm so lucky to be one of them. So far there have been a few remissions. That's exciting."

"How does it work, Hirshel?"

"The doctors don't know for sure. Somehow it employs the body's own defense system. My specialist thinks the drug unleashes your body's natural killer cells so they can attack and destroy the cancer cells. They're trying it on a lot of other cancers and even multiple sclerosis and AIDS. It might even get rid of colds. It's real space-age stuff.

"They make it in a laboratory from recombinant DNA. It's extremely expensive to produce. Thank God research volunteers like me don't have to pay for it. It's amazing what scientists can do today, but it's scary too. . . . I wonder what the Talmudic rabbis would say about this, Jim. Do you think they'd allow it? Isn't genetic engineering tampering with nature?"

"I think they'd approve if it helps people and saves lives, don't you? Nature is created by God as we were. We have to take care of our environment, but we can use our God-given intelligence to improve on it. Genetic engineering is just one of the new issues we have to deal with, like organ transplants and test-tube babies. There are so many ethical dilemmas involved. Change is part of life, and it will always pose problems and questions and challenges.

"You know, Hirshel, right before my brother died I heard about an experimental treatment for cancer called transfer factor. I phoned around the country desperately and finally tracked down the doctor in charge of the program. I convinced Bert's physicians to get it and try it on him, which wasn't easy. I think it did help him. He became much more alert, and maybe it gave him an extra few weeks of life. I wonder if that transfer factor was the same thing as interferon. Maybe if Bert had become sick now instead of eleven years ago, he could have been saved. But what's the point of dwelling on that? I'm just glad it's available for you now."

Three weeks later Hirshel phones to tell me they got the hospital bill from Chicago. "It's just staggering, Jim. You can't even imagine how much it is. The cheapest thing on the bill cost eight dollars. That was for Tylenol! It's a good thing we have some financial help. There's really something wrong with our medical system in this country. What do poor people who get sick do? Sometimes the private hospitals won't even take them.

"I met a patient in the Chicago hospital who has my disease, and we had a long talk one night. Before he got sick he had a high income. Suddenly his family was financially devastated. They had never envisioned what could happen. He's consumed by the fact that he won't be able to send his children to college. I try not to become obsessed with finances. There's only one thing that really counts now. It's very simple—I have to try to survive, or nothing else matters."

"How are you feeling, Hirshel?"

"The fevers are getting scary. I have them almost all the time now, and last Friday I had to stop conducting services. Sometimes they get up to 103 and 104. Once I had almost 105, and I was nearly delirious. Judi was up most of the night with me. It's like I'm in the hospital and she's my nurse. It isn't fair to her. The fevers debilitate me so I can't get out of bed much. And I've lost a lot of weight.

"My doctors are really worried, and they're just stumped. One of them admitted, 'Medical science just doesn't know enough about your bizarre disease.' They still think the fevers might be caused by that rare tuberculosis, but nothing is showing up on the X-rays or the cultures."

Hirshel continues to have the high fevers for several more weeks. Now they reach almost 105 degrees, and Judi is frantic. The doctors seem immobilized. Finally, one day when Marcia telephones the Jaffes, there's no answer. She tries all day. We're worried because Hirshel is always at home except for brief visits to his doctors. That night we get a call from Stephanie Goldstein. She's also worried because she can't locate Hirshel and Judi. We agree to telephone each other if either of us hears anything.

The next day Stephanie phones to tell us she has found out Hirshel is back in the Chicago hospital. He's undergoing lung surgery.

"The local doctor suddenly found something on a chest X-ray and heard a strange, crackling noise in his breathing," Judi explains when she finally gets a chance to telephone us from Chicago. "They took out a piece of his lung to culture it and see if it's that rare TB. They did the surgery on the first night of Chanukkah. I handed Hirshel a Chanukkah card from the kids right before they wheeled him down to the operating room.

"They can't be absolutely sure it's that tuberculosis until the culture of his biopsy grows out, but the doctors are betting that's what's giving him the fevers. That might also be the source of his mysterious cough. They're starting him on a variety of anti-TB drugs to try to knock it out. He's taking thirteen pills a day, plus some injections. It's terribly powerful stuff. The pills are so big I don't see how he can even swallow them."

"He's getting all that other medicine on top of the interferon, and they're not even sure he has this tuberculosis?" I ask.

"That's right. But this infection is so dangerous they have to try everything they can to stop it. They shouldn't have let the fevers go on this long. They're ravaging his body. Sometimes his chills are so bad the nurses have to give him injections to stop him from shaking. He could barely walk when I took him out to Chicago, and his breathing was very shallow. Apparently the blood cells weren't carrying enough oxygen to his body. I was afraid he'd die on the airplane. He's a bag of bones, too. I kept trying to tell his doctors he's losing too much weight, and they kept telling me how good his blood counts are because of the interferon. They were elated about them. When we got to Chicago I said, 'Stop reading the damned blood counts and look at your patient! He's not looking too good!'

"Now he's in pain and weak from the surgery. He's

lost thirty pounds at least. His weight went down into the one-thirties. He won't eat, so they're feeding him through an IV. I keep trying to get him to eat something, but he has to force himself."

After Judi goes back to Newburgh, we telephone Hirshel every day. But most of the time we get a busy signal.

"I'm sorry, but I've been leaving the phone off the hook," Hirshel whispers in a weak voice when we finally get through to him. "I just didn't feel like talking to anybody."

"Are you eating anything?" Marcia nags.

"Can't, I don't want to. Judi got exasperated with me when she was here. One day she knew she had to jar me, so she said, 'OK, Hirshel, if you aren't going to eat I'm going to go shopping,' and she left for the rest of the afternoon. I ate something just to show her. I'm not getting out of bed and moving around like I'm supposed to, either. I'm too weak. And I just found out I'll have to take these antibiotics for a year or more because this tuberculosis strain is so difficult to get rid of. But they're saving my life.

"I'm lonely here without Judi, but I understand why she had to go home. A few of our Chicago colleagues are popping in to see me, and Judi's wonderful aunt who lives here visits me all the time. My cousin flew out and surprised me. And my parents keep calling. I wish they would come out here, but I know they're still having trouble coping."

Either Marcia or I telephone Hirshel every day, though we almost dread calling because we don't know how he'll be. One day he's so weak he can barely speak, the next day his voice sounds stronger and he feels better, and the following day he's weak and depressed again. And yet somehow he manages to keep his spirits up and to keep going in his endless battle. We wonder where he gets his inner strength. But Marcia and I are having trouble keeping *our* spirits up.

One day at a luncheon one of my friends, a very religious Christian minister, tells me I'm looking "down." I tell him Hirshel's story.

"But surely as a rabbi doesn't he have faith in an afterlife?" my friend tries to console me.

"Well, it's not quite so simple. Judaism is vague when it comes to describing precisely what life after death is like. Perhaps it would be easier for us to face this ordeal if we did have a clearer idea. I know it would make our jobs as rabbis much easier. When I officiate at funerals, the family often asks what our religion teaches about afterlife. They want to be told something concrete, something that will console them.

"We do believe in the immortality of the soul," I explain to my friend, "but our ideas about the afterlife aren't systematized, and they've varied at different times throughout our history. You know, the Hebrew Bible doesn't say anything about an immortal soul or a world to come. It implies that behavior is rewarded or punished in *this* life. The Bible does mention Sheol, the Valley of Gehinnom, a hill outside the old city in Jerusalem where they threw garbage and waste and bodies of animals and criminals. But we don't know much about it except that it's a dark and shadowy place, a pit underneath the earth separated from our world, where there is no God. In the Bible, and for later Jews too, punishment is a life without God.

"Around the first century B.C.E. we developed various ideas about a separate soul surviving the body, physical resurrection of the body after death, and a Messiah—a king of Israel who will usher in the final age of peace and justice, when everyone will stand before God for judgment. The early Christians inherited these concepts from Judaism and made them part of their new religion.

"Talmudic scholars thought of eternal life as *Olam Haba*, the 'World to Come,' a place where all righteous souls will dwell eternally with God. They believed the great sages will sit in a semicircle in a heavenly scholarly academy with God presiding at the helm. The rabbis compared afterlife to what we value on earth. The joy of eternal life, for example, is like the pleasure a student gets from studying Torah. Since the Sabbath, the day of rest, is one of life's great joys, eternity is like a long 'day that is all Sabbath.'

"One Talmudic rabbi said this world is like a foyer leading to the World to Come. We should prepare ourselves in the foyer before entering the inner chamber. But others didn't want the vision of divine reward or punishment to overshadow the importance of living a good life for its own sake. This ambiguity is summarized by a scholar who said, 'Richer is one hour of repentance and good works in this world than all of life in the world to come; and richer is one hour's calm of spirit in the world to come than all of life in this world.'

"In the Middle Ages some Jewish mystics believed in transmigration, reincarnation, of the soul. . . ."

"I didn't know there were Jewish mystics!" my friend interrupts.

"Oh, yes, we have a long mystical tradition which culminated in the Hassidic movement in Europe in the eighteenth century. They believed the soul has a task to complete and it wanders from life to life until it finishes its job on earth and ascends to God. A bad person's soul is doomed to wander forever. The mystics thought of eternity as spiritual bliss, outside of time, a state of mind, rather than an actual place.

"Of course our great Jewish philosophers conjectured

about the soul's immortality. Maimonides basically thought of the world to come as pure spirit. But most Jewish philosophers warned against speculating too much about afterlife. They felt it was useless."

"And today what do Jews believe?" my Christian friend asks.

"Well, traditional Jews believe in physical resurrection of the body. That's why they're opposed to autopsies, organ donations, and cremation—the body must be intact for the resurrection, which will take place when the Messiah arrives and brings on the Last Days, the Day of Judgment. Then the graves will open and everyone will be judged and rewarded.

"Liberal Jews look forward to a Messianic Age, rather than to a specific person. This will be a time of social justice. It's an ongoing human goal to strive for rather than an eschatological concept. We don't believe in resurrection of the body, but we believe the human spirit transcends death and all souls will dwell with God. All Jews feel people live on in the memories of their children and the others who loved them, and through the good works they leave behind on earth."

The Jewish tradition emphasizes that finding God in this life is reward enough, so promise of eternal life as a reward should not be necessary, I explain to my friend. We perform the *Mitzvot*, our commandments, because they bring joy in this life, not so we'll be rewarded in an afterlife. According to an eighteenth-century folk tale, the founder of the Hassidic movement, Israel ben Eliezer, known as the Baal Shem Tov, once became so depressed that he thought, "I have no share in the world to come." Then he said to himself, "If I love God, what need have I of paradise?" When someone asked Rabbi Eliezer how to attain eternal life, he replied, "Show concern for the honor of your friends; set your children at the feet of the wise, who will keep them from idle thoughts; and, when you pray, know before whom you stand. Thus will you win eternal life."

Death is inevitable, and we must accept its reality. But we shouldn't dwell on it and let it detract from the value of *this* life. Ironically, or perhaps appropriately, the Kaddish, the Jewish prayer recited in memory of the dead, says nothing about death. Instead it affirms life by praising and glorifying God and His creation.

Even Judaism's mourning rituals are life-oriented. After someone dies, we must grieve fully, acknowledging the sadness and the reality of death—which certainly fits in well with contemporary psychological theory. But the highly organized mourning rituals are designed to channel our grief and return the bereaved to active life and a positive state of mind as soon as possible.

There is a period called *Shivah* (the Hebrew word for "seven"), when we stay at home for seven days to receive condolence calls from comforting family and friends. Even children must "sit *Shivah*" so they, too, can face the reality of death and be part of this meaningful family ritual. At the end of that time we resume a normal schedule except for a thirty-day period when we avoid going to places of entertainment, and we recite memorial prayers daily. Then the immediate family continues its prayers for the deceased for eleven months.

After that time we are forbidden to dwell on the death and must attempt to reenter life fully. "Do not abandon yourself to grief," counsels the Wisdom of Ben Sira. "Put it from you and think of your own end. . . . Remember that his fate will also be yours. . . . When the dead is at rest, let his memory rest too."

When reform rabbis compiled a new prayer book in the 1970s, they included a poem by Rabbi Alvin Fine in the High Holiday liturgy. It is one of my favorites, not only because it is so beautiful, but because it expresses an idea with which I agree—that life is a journey of constant growth. Living itself is its own reward, and eternal life is a process, not a product.

> Birth is a beginning
> And death a destination.
> And life is a journey:
> From childhood to maturity
> And youth to age;
> From innocence to awareness
> And ignorance to knowing;
> From foolishness to discretion
> And then, perhaps, to wisdom;
> From weakness to strength
> Or strength to weakness—
> And, often, back again;
> From health to sickness
> And back, we pray, to health again;
> From offense to forgiveness,
> From loneliness to love,
> From joy to gratitude,
> From pain to compassion,
> And grief to understanding—
> From fear to faith;
> From defeat to defeat to defeat—
> Until, looking backward or ahead,
> We see that victory lies
> Not at some high place along the way,
> But in having made the journey, stage by stage,
> A sacred pilgrimage.
> Birth is a beginning
> And death a destination.
> And life is a journey,
> A sacred pilgrimage—
> To life everlasting.

I've passed another hurdle. I'm able to eat again. Not much, but enough to start gaining some strength back and so the nurses can disconnect the IV from my arm. I'm trying to move around and walk up and down the halls. But now I have a new problem. I had a bad reaction to one of the TB drugs, and I have a lot of pain when I try to walk. It hurts to put my feet on the floor. My right hand is arthritic too. They're giving me pills to ease the pain. One more drug going into my body . . .

The doctors hope if they take me off the antibiotics and reintroduce them one by one they'll discover the culprit. They aren't sure why I'm having this terrible joint pain. They say I'm one for the medical books. I tell them I always was a troublemaker! The doctors are agonizing over me, and that's a comfort. I know they even kept telephoning the specialist about my case when he was at a hematology conference in Florida.

My congregants finally hired a very nice, retired rabbi part-time to fill in for me. Judi told me so many people back in Newburgh are in the dark about my condition that rumors are spreading through my congregation again as they did when I was in the hospital for so long after my spleenectomy. They're saying I'm not coming back, that I'm going to die out here. But I'm going to pull through! If they can lick this tuberculosis and the interferon works, then I've got a chance. . . .

Christmas.
Last night a group of carolers came through our halls. The singing got louder as they came nearer to me, and I was touched because of what they were doing for the other patients.

When they came to my door, they suddenly starting singing *Chanukkah* songs. The last night of *Chanukkah* coincides with Christmas this year, and they heard I was a rabbi. I sang along with them. Later Judi came to my room, and we lit all eight candles on a little *Chanukkah* menorah she brought. She held my hand to steady it and helped me light the last candle.

Today one of the young carolers, a hospital volunteer, came back and told me she's Jewish and so was the guy dressed up as Santa Claus. She said when we sang *Chanukkah* songs in my room last night she finally understood what it means for Christians to hear Christmas carols at this time of year. She told me it meant a lot to her to be singing *Chanukkah* songs with a rabbi.

December 27, 1984

I was finally able to call Rachel and Nina on the telephone. Before today it's just been too much for me to talk to them. I was afraid I'd break down.

My girls are having a great vacation from school. They go skiing nearly every day. Judi is bringing them out to see me over the long New Year's weekend. I need them close to me so much.

My parents flew out to Chicago today. It was a very emotional visit. I'm glad I had some good news for them. My chest X-rays are looking better, so those strong antibiotics must be doing something to stop the infection. The doctors probably guessed correctly—I must have that strange TB because my fevers seem to be disappearing. I'm even coughing less, so they think maybe the cough was caused by the TB. Finally I'm gaining back some weight. And my blood counts are still going up dramatically because of the interferon, so at last I'm not in such mortal danger of infection. The doctors are thrilled with my progress.

They're starting to talk about when I'm going home. Judi sent me my good blue Adidas running suit to wear when I work out in the physical training room downstairs. The doctors say I need this therapy and I should ride on the exercise bike down there. I'm weak now, but they tell me if I exercise I'll build up my strength again.

It'll be great to go home. But, strangely, it will be hard to say good-bye to everyone here. The hospital becomes your entire world, the people who care for you, especially the other patients. And the doctors and I have gotten fond of each other. We know about each other's families.

I've regained so much esteem for the medical profession. I know I'm not just another theoretical medical case to these doctors. One said, "Rabbi Jaffe, you're another example of living proof that interferon can work." It's powerful; it's very exciting to them. I realize these wonderful physicians and I are standing together at an uncharted frontier of science. We've plunged into this endeavor together, inexorably linked. Instead of the frequent doctor-patient one-upmanship situation, we're real partners, and that's good for my battered morale.

Today my specialist came into my room. He said I am definitely entering a period of remission again! I could hardly believe it! I thought he just wanted to talk about my future medical treatment, but then he sat down. He seemed so earnest and intense. He told me I had so much to offer people with this disease, that I have almost a mission to encourage them and give them hope.

I was flattered, and at first I thought he was just trying to make me feel good. But I could tell by his eyes that he was sincere. He asked me if he could give other hairy-cell leukemia patients my address and telephone number so they can get in touch with me for counseling.

Of course I said yes. How could I do less? I know how important it is to talk about your feelings. It's gratifying to think I can help others. It's a way of giving back something, of showing my thanks because I've been spared. And if I can use my experience to help others going through the same thing, my struggle will have meaning.

But just as I was feeling so good about myself, I began to wonder if God isn't maybe being a little capricious after all. One physician told me if they'd let my fevers go another week I would have died. My specialist just happened to remember this strange tuberculosis. He saved my life. It was really a rush against time. And without this interferon I would be a goner. But if I'd needed it last year instead of this year I wouldn't have been able to get it, because they just started this inter-feron program. It's really just an accident that I fit their requirements for acceptance into the program.

And it's another accident that I got this disease when I did. They hadn't even identified hairy-cell leukemia until recently. Previously they mistook it for other kinds of leukemia and gave the wrong treatment and people died. And they've only just begun to understand it in the last few years. That almost makes me feel guilty. I ask myself, "Why should I have a chance for survival when somebody else a few years ago didn't even have that chance?" It's like being born in America instead of in Europe during the Holocaust, surviving Hitler because of geography.

And why should I be able to go home now and be with my family when other patients are stuck in this hospital?

I've become very close to a young man I met in the physical therapy room. He's confined to his wheelchair. Last night he wheeled himself into my doorway. He was all bundled up in a sweat shirt and blankets because his cancer gives him con-stant chills. We were getting ourselves ready to part company —we know how tough it's going to be—and we exchanged addresses and made small talk. He said, "I'm happy that you'll be going home soon, Hirshel." But I knew that he's aching to go home too, and I could see the pain in his eyes.

I said, "I'll miss you," and I tried to make a joke, but I couldn't. Our eyes just locked together in a long gaze. It was very emotional.

Finally he spun his wheelchair around and said weakly, "I have to go back to my room now," and wheeled himself away as fast as he could. I turned away from the door and shouted out, "Dammit, why does a good kid like that have to suffer?"

December 31, 1984

It's New Year's Eve. The snow is coming down rapidly outside my window.

I got a beautiful card from one of the women in my congregation today. In it she wrote, "It's Shabbat and the house is snug and cozy against the sleet falling outside. My thoughts are miles away, with you, wishing you strength and energy so that like a modern-day Maccabee you may win your battle in sure triumph. I cast off those somber clouds and send you April and sunshine and sparrow songs and gentle breezes. . . . Look out your window and see the rainbow stretching from Newburgh to Chicago, from all of us to you, and reminding you as God did Noah that with it we send our love."

This is the kind of love and support that enables me to keep up this battle. . . .

I'm so happy that Judi and Rachel and Nina are here with me tonight for New Year's Eve. They arrived yesterday. It's been so long since I've seen them, and I have missed them very much.

Everybody on the floor knows Judi, of course. She was by my side for endless hours after I had the lung surgery, and she stayed late every night and got close to the nurses. One night Judi ordered a big pizza and force-fed it to the nurses. So naturally Judi planned a party for everyone on the floor tonight for New Year's Eve. She bought some Sangria and white wine, and the kids brought in soda and cookies and potato chips.

The nurses are sipping wine and all the patients who can make it are down in the lounge. The TV set is turned up loud so we'll be ready for the countdown at midnight. Some people are singing. Judi has been coaxing me to have some Sangria too. I feel so good I think I will have a little to toast the new year.

Nineteen eighty-five. A new year. A fresh start.

February 8, 1985

It's like a miracle. I'm back in my temple for Sabbath services. I'm still getting my strength back, so the temporary rabbi will officiate. But I'll sit on the pulpit with him, and I'll recite a special Hebrew prayer of thanksgiving for my recovery.

I searched the liturgy and found a prayer that could have been written just for me: "O God, for the grave illness through which I have recently passed, I thank You. All life is in Your hands, and You have spared me. Let me show my gratitude by learning to welcome each day with thanks. Let me learn to devote my life to sharing it with my loved ones and with those who seek me in their need. Praise be to God, Ruler of the universe, who has granted to me much good."

March 22, 1985

In a few minutes I officially return to my job. The fill-in rabbi has left, and now it's up to me to lead Sabbath services. It's been so long since I've been in charge I'm nervous, almost like a beginner.

I'm sitting in my study going over the service and trying to collect my thoughts.

I really worked hard on my sermon for tonight. I'm trying to relate it to what I've gone through with this illness. My people want to know what I've learned from this experience, if I have discovered meaning in my suffering. I'm going to tell them yes, I have. I've struggled with my leukemia and agonized and asked, "Why me?" and raged at the pain it's brought me. But I can't agree with those who say it's all meaningless; I couldn't survive if I believed that. So I have searched for meaning. It isn't easy, but you have to find meaning in life and in suffering because you can't live without hope and purpose.

I'll begin my sermon tonight with that famous, moving story about a group of Jewish physicians incarcerated in the Buchenwald concentration camp. They went through the same horrors as everybody else, but they set goals for themselves. Every night when all the other prisoners were asleep these exhausted doctors met secretly. As if they were still in practice they discussed medical cases of the camp inmates, and prepared and presented scholarly papers to each other.

Then the doctors began to smuggle materials into the camp so they could build medical instruments. I don't know how they did it—bribed the guards, hid the stolen pieces in their clothes. Eventually with the help of other prisoners who were engineers and electricians they were able to construct an X-ray machine that worked. They used it at night secretly to diagnose sick prisoners. I'll tell my congregation these physicians accomplished this miracle because they never lost hope or their sense of purpose.

Then I'll talk about a book I read years ago written by psychiatrist Victor Frankl, who went through the Nazi concentration camps and lost almost all his family in the Holocaust.

While Frankl was in Dachau and Auschwitz, he devised a goal, a purpose for himself. He decided to observe people scientifically to see how they were reacting to their horrible dehumanizing experiences in the camps. He could see that

191

different people reacted differently to the same circumstances of immense suffering. He observed that how they reacted determined to a large extent whether or not they survived their ordeal.

Frankl discovered that the people who survived Hitler's death camps were those like himself who had set a purpose for themselves. Their positive attitude helped them interpret tragic circumstances differently from other victims, helped them triumph over the circumstances rather than be overcome by them. Frankl says we can't always choose our circumstances or suffering, but we can and must choose how we are going to react to the circumstances and suffering. No matter what our experiences or fate, we are free to choose our attitude *toward the experiences, toward life. So we can find meaning and hope even in the darkest of days.*

I didn't choose *my illness; I didn't ask for this painful experience. But I can choose my attitude toward it; I can forge my own response to it. Since it* is *happening to me, I can choose to make the best of it; I can use it and learn from it and grow from it, shape it into a positive force in my life.*

I've definitely been transformed through this experience. I've learned how vulnerable we are, that our lives are in God's hands. I know what's really important now. We should be thankful for each day granted us, and greet it joyously. Now I fully enjoy every aspect of my life. Every moment is special to me.

And I know this illness has transformed every aspect of my work. I know I am a better rabbi. People always tell me I have so much more spiritual depth now. I think these new spiritual resources got me through my struggle. This seems to inspire people. My example seems to give them courage to face their own problems.

Before I left the hospital in Chicago, my specialist used the word "mission" when he asked me to counsel other hairy-cell leukemia patients. That made me realize I do have a special task. Maybe I had to undergo this illness in order to help people better and in that way serve God. Maybe that's God's purpose for me. Maybe that is the meaning of my struggle.

Since I became sick I think about Psalm 138 all the time because it expresses this thought so beautifully. A calligraphy version of that psalm given to me by a friend hangs on my study wall here in the temple. I find myself constantly glancing up at it now because it has become so meaningful to me:

When I called to Thee Thou didst answer me and make me bold and valiant hearted. . . . With Thy right hand thou savest me. The Lord will accomplish His purpose for me. Thy true love, O Lord, endures forever; leave not Thy work unfinished.

The cantor just knocked on my study door. It's time for the service to begin.